VEGAN DIET
for
ATHLETES and
BODYBUILDERS

How to Build Muscle
and Gain Weight

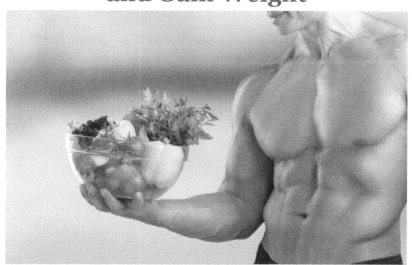

with Plant-Based Food?

Table of Content

What is a Vegan?

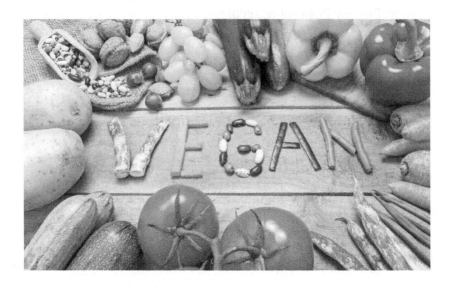

The origins of vegetarianism date back to ancient times. But the term «Vegan» was first used in the 40s by Donald Watson, co-founder of the Vegan Society, to describe a lifestyle doctrine that man should live without exploiting animals.

The following decades saw substantial growth in the industrialization of food production and an increase in the nature of food. We seemed to move from a "garden to plate" life to a 'factory to plate". Food came out of convenient packets, which we threw away after eating the unhealthy contents, resulting in bad health for us and garbage and gasses for the planet.

By the 70s attitudes to health followed a trend toward a more natural lifestyle. Cultures blended many ideas from the East, and food production in western countries came under scrutiny. Along with a movement towards more compassionate living, people started to become critical of meat-eating and the way animals are treated when they are bred for food.

A move towards more natural food production methods for plants and animals started gaining awareness amongst the younger generations, who had to deal with the damage that unhealthy food production was causing to the earth, to plants and animals, and us.

Vegetarianism became a trend a growing trend in the west. But also, we now realize that some cultures have been traditionally vegetarian for thousands of years.

Veganism seems to have evolved from recognizing that even a vegetarian lifestyle still doesn't improve the risk of certain kinds of health issues and that even a vegetarian lifestyle doesn't eliminate the suffering caused to animals when they are used for what they produce. Vegetarianism has become a trend in the West. But also, we now realize that some cultures have been traditionally vegetarian for thousands of years.

The production of eggs still involves the battery farming of chickens. Cows are physically restrained for hours a day, not to mention the diet and medical intervention required to make them produce more milk than they are evolved to produce.

Veganism recognizes that any treatment of animals that raises them for the production of food and products involves some measure of suffering.

We will look at more specific aspects of veganism and a vegan dietary choice in this book.

Types of Vegetarianism and their differences

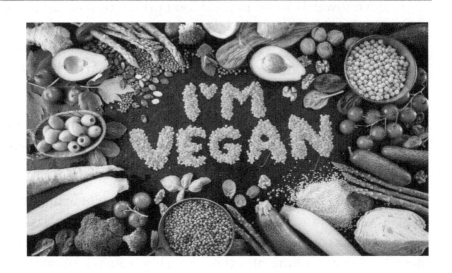

Veganism and vegetarianism - just words or a way of life?

People often do not understand the difference between vegans and vegetarians.

The reason is that the very concept of vegetarianism is inaccurate and can mean different eating styles. Vegetarianism (from Lat. Vegetarius - vegetable) is a common name for food systems (diets) based on the use of plant products and the exclusion or limitation of the consumption of animal products.

Veganism is a lifestyle based on great moral awareness. The diet itself is only a consequence of the moral and ethical views of veganism. Vegans have special dietary rules, and veganism is often practiced for ethical reasons. Below we look at vegan principles in more detail.

Types of vegetarianism:

> Lacto-ovo-vegetarianism
> Lacto-vegetarianism
> Ovo-vegetarianism
> Veganism
> Raw food diet
> Fruitarianism
> Unusual types of vegetarian diets (Polotarianism, Pescatarism)

Lacto-ovo-vegetarianism

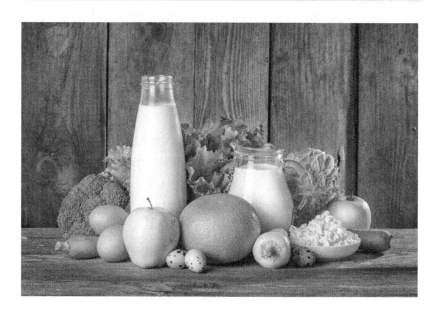

In the modern world, Lacto-ovo-vegetarianism can be called the most common vegetarian diet.

The term Lacto-ovo-vegetarianism itself comes from Latin words: lacto - milk, egg - egg, vegetation - vegetation.

As the name implies, a lacto-ovo-vegetarian diet allows you to use milk and dairy products, eggs and any plant products.

Any meat of animals, whether it is meat, poultry, fish or seafood, is excluded from the diet.

As followers of any other vegetarian diet, lacto-ovo-vegetarians are divided into ethical vegetarians who adhere to the vegetarian diet for ethical or religious reasons, and vegetarians who adhere to this diet for the benefit of their health.

If your diet is balanced correctly, then switching to a lacto-ovo-vegetarian diet will be completely painless for you. The fact is that animal products will remain on your daily menu. You can still eat egg and dairy products. Almost all your favorite dishes may well remain on your menu.

A properly planned lacto-ovo-vegetarian diet should include the following products weekly:

6-12 servings of cereal products, cereals, legumes
6-8 servings of dairy products (cheese, milk, cottage cheese, natural yogurt, sour cream, etc.)
4-6 servings of vegetables and vegetable dishes
3-5 servings of fruit
1-2 eggs per day (including eggs that are already found in various foods, such as baked goods).

It is also recommended that you include nuts and dried fruits in your diet. Nuts contain a large amount of protein, phosphorus, zinc, magnesium, iron, calcium, and dried fruits are an excellent source of iron.

Lacto-vegetarianism

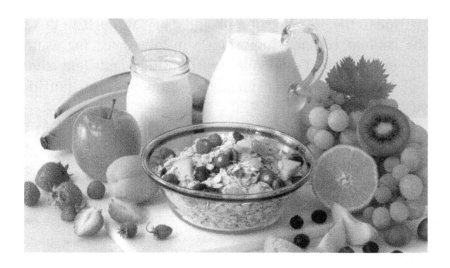

The word "Lacto-vegetarianism" consists of two parts. The prefix «lacto-» comes from the Latin word "lactis", which means milk. The second part - vegetarianism - is well known to everyone who is at least to some extent interested in the problem of healthy eating.

It is also the most popular course among vegetarians.

Lacto-vegetarianism is a vegetarian diet that, in addition to vegetable products, allows you to consume milk and dairy products, whether it is cheese, cottage cheese, butter, etc. But lacto-vegetarians may not eat all kinds of cheeses. Cheeses that contain an enzyme of animal origin, such as abomasum, are excluded from the diet.

Lacto-vegetarians exclude from their diet all products of animal origin, including eggs, only dairy products are allowed. Dairy products in this form of nutrition are the main source of protein.

To a large extent, lacto-vegetarianism is ethical vegetarianism. People on this diet believe that products of animal origin can be used, but only if they are obtained by non-violent means.

Due to the presence of milk and dairy products in this diet, the content of such important substances as, for example, calcium, vitamin D and vitamin B12, will be sufficient, and you will not need to consume large amounts of nutritional supplements.

Also, thanks to dairy products, you can be sure that your body receives all the necessary amino acids.

Ovo-vegetarianism

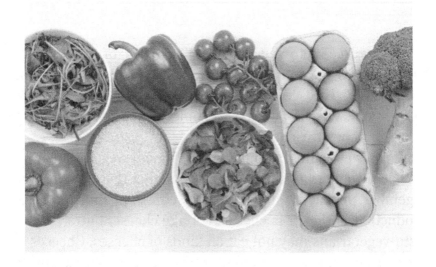

Ovo-vegetarianism is a type of vegetarianism excluding all animal products except eggs.

Like lacto-vegetarians, ovo-vegetarians are convinced of the need to eat animal protein and, in particular, an egg.

But there is one important point - you can eat only unfertilized eggs. If the eggs are fertilized, then a new life has already begun in it, which cannot be killed.

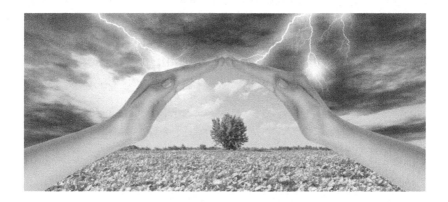

People who are, or have been vegetarian for a long time, think switching to Veganism is easy. After all, you have not eaten meat or animal products for ages. Then you reach for the honey to sweeten your tea and realize that the vegan life means no honey or milk in that steaming mug of tea.

So honey is a "No", but what about silk from silkworms or makeup using animal by-products?

Veganism is a lifestyle based on great moral mindfulness. The diet itself is only a consequence of the moral and ethical views of veganism.

Veganism as a diet has a very large ethical component. This is the case when people are primarily guided by humane and moral considerations.

Veganism is to live in harmony with nature and the world around us, to understand ourselves as a part of this nature.

This also includes refusing fishing and hunting, a circus where animals work, and zoos, and everything else where there is at least a hint of unnatural treatment of animals.

Vegans absolutely exclude from the diet all products of animal origin, even seemingly innocent honey, since this is a product of exploitation. These people do not wear any fur products and clothes of all kinds of leather. Vegans use only cosmetics, the production of which did not use components of animal origin, as well as in the production process, which were not carried out on animals. Veganism is often called the extreme form of vegetarianism, although this is not entirely true. An extreme form of vegetarianism, rather, should be called a raw food diet.

Raw food diet

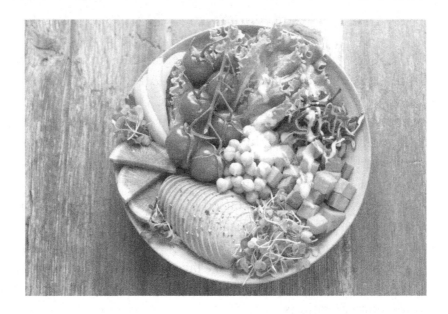

A raw food diet is a food system in which foods are consumed that did not go through any kind of heat treatment in the kitchen, such as stewing, baking, frying, smoke-dry, and others. It is believed that with this method of nutrition, the nutritional value of the products is fully preserved.

Raw foodists exclude from the diet of all products of animal origin and really eat exclusively raw vegetables and fruits. Food is never cooked. It is allowed to dry in the sun or in the oven at a temperature of no higher than 42 degrees. The list of allowed foods for raw foodists includes fresh fruits and vegetables, cereals, dried fruits, nuts, berries, herbs, germinate various cereal seeds and all kinds of cold-pressed oils.

Fruitarianism

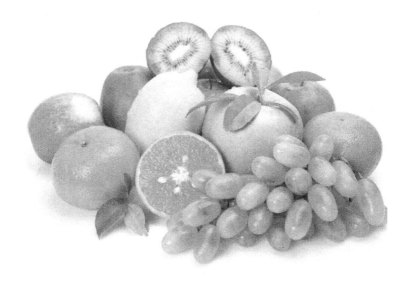

Eating fruit is probably the sweetest type of raw food diet.

Fruitarians themselves define their diet as a diet with a predominant content of raw fruits in the diet (from 75 to 100% of the diet), sometimes with the addition of some other vegetarian foods (more often nuts and seeds, less often some vegetables). Some of the strictest followers of the Fruitarian diet eat only those fruits and nuts that themselves fell from the trees, explaining this by the desire not to participate in the killing of any living creatures, including plants.

However, the balance of such a diet is subject to great doubt by well-known nutritionists.

Scientists from the University of Columbia (Columbia University in the City of New York) have proved that a fruitarian diet leads to a serious deficiency in the human body of substances such as protein, calcium, iron, zinc, vitamin D, most B vitamins (especially B12) and essential fatty acids.

Short-term dietary courses based on Fruitarianism can be considered as diet options for those who want to lose weight or seek to cleanse the body. But it should be remembered that even extreme diets, such as fruitarianism, can only be followed for a short time after consulting a nutritionist, and in the presence of any serious illnesses, only after consulting a doctor.

Polotarianism

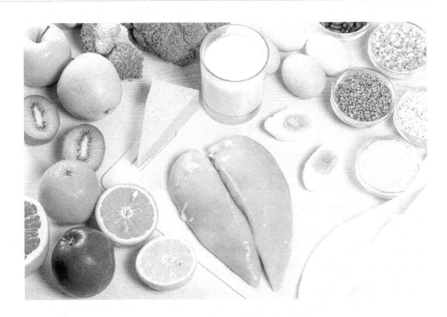

Polotarianism (pollotarianism) is an unusual type of vegetarian diet. This diet excludes the consumption of meat of animal type mammals (red meat). In this case, it is allowed to eat poultry meat, fish, eggs, milk.

Pescetarism

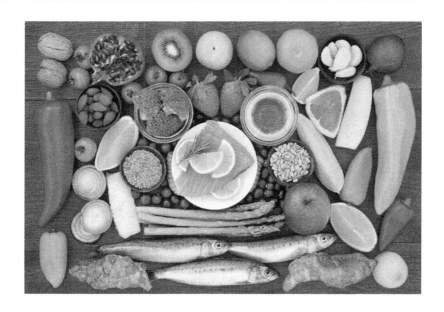

Pescetarism - from the word pesce or pescado, which means "fish" - is an unusual type of vegetarian diet too. This diet allows you to eat fish and seafood. Dairy products and eggs usually are not consumed. However, 70-80% of the diet consists of vegetables, herbs, cereals, and legumes. Fish and seafood in the diet play only the role of an additional source of protein. A pescetarian diet is similar to a traditional Mediterranean diet. Like the Mediterranean diet, a healthy pescetarian diet consists of lots of fruits and vegetables, whole grains, nuts, and legumes. This diet is quite flexible. In addition, most pescetarians, like vegetarians, leave dairy products and eggs in their diets.

Plant-based diet vs Veganism vs Vegetarianism - what's the difference?

Veganism vs Plant-based diet

A plant-based diet is based on plant-based foods and is virtually no different from a vegan diet in terms of nutrition. It's just a nutritional style of plant-based foods for maintaining and improving health.

Veganism is not only a plant-based diet but also a special ethical lifestyle. Strict veganism is to live in harmony with nature and the world, to protect all kinds of animals and stop any exploitation of creatures that live next to us on our planet. Most vegans decide to follow this diet for cultural, ethical, or religious reasons.

Vegans try to avoid all forms of cruelty too, and exploitation of animals for food, clothing, or any other purpose. This doesn't necessarily infer that vegans consume lots of wholefood meals, they can consume processed foods and snub their veggies. Just like anyone else, they can consume (vegan-friendly) gummy candy, potato chips and even cookies.

A plant-based diet, on the other hand, places more emphasis on consuming whole fruits and vegetables, eating lots of whole grains, and avoiding or minimizing the consumption of processed foods or animal products for health reasons. There are no definitions or strict guidelines for what makes up a plant-based diet other than placing emphasis on the consumption of fresh produce and eating a minimal quantity of processed foods.

The main difference is that different types of vegetarians can eat some products of animal origin (milk, cheese, eggs, sometimes even fish or poultry). We talked about this in detail above. A plant-based diet consists solely of plant-based foods and focuses on the consumption of fresh produce and eating a minimal quantity of processed foods. And any products of animal origin are excluded.

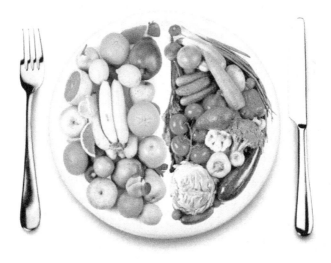

The health benefits of the Vegan diet

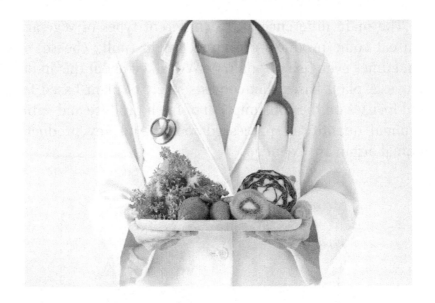

In nations and populations following a traditional vegetarian diet like many eastern cultures, the incidence of lifestyle diseases like heart disease and diabetes, or the kinds of diseases we usually develop from a lifetime of over-indulgence, is very low or had been before some cultures started adopting a more western eating pattern.

All the evidence, and there is too much to present in this book, seems to say that vegetarian, and especially plant-only based diets are the best protection we can give ourselves against lifestyle diseases and cancers.

So, the health benefits of the vegan diet:

Better Nutrition

Plants are very healthy foods to eat and most people fail to eat the appropriate amount of veggies and fruits, therefore, following a plant-based diet will boost your productivity, and this is a very nutritious option. Vegetables and fruits are rich in antioxidants, vitamins, fibers, and minerals. Based on studies, fiber is known to be a nutrient that most people don't get an adequate amount of, and it comes with tons of healthy perks—is good for the heart, waistline, blood sugar and the gut. However, science also shows that overall nutrition is better when following a vegan or vegetarian diet versus when following an omnivorous diet.

Weight loss

When following a vegan diet you tend to gain a lower body mass index (BMI) compared to people on an omnivorous diet. However, research shows that when you follow a vegetarian diet in order to lose weight, you will be more successful at dropping pounds, and also keeping them off.

Healthier hearts

Following a vegetarian diet is likely to reduce the risk of cardiovascular diseases, and enhance other risk factors for heart disease by reducing cholesterol, and blood pressure, and enhancing the blood sugar control.

Lower diabetes risk

Irrespective of your body mass index (BMI), following a vegan diet or a vegetarian diet, lowers the risk of diabetes. However, a study shows that people who eat meat have a higher risk of diabetes compared to Lacto-ovo vegans and vegetarians. Another study, published in February 2019, states that when you follow a vegetarian diet, you tend to have a higher insulin sensitivity; this is significant for maintaining a healthy blood sugar level.

Reduces the risk of cancer

The consistent consumption of adequate legumes, veggies, fruits, and grains is associated with a lower cancer risk. However, disease-fighting phytochemicals that can be found in plants are known to prevent and halt cancer. Lastly, studies also indicate an association between the consumption of processed meats and a rise in the risk of cancer, especially colorectal cancer. Therefore, there's a benefit not just from the consumption of more plants, but also from choosing healthy plant foods rather than unhealthy ones.

How to become a vegetarian without harm to the body?

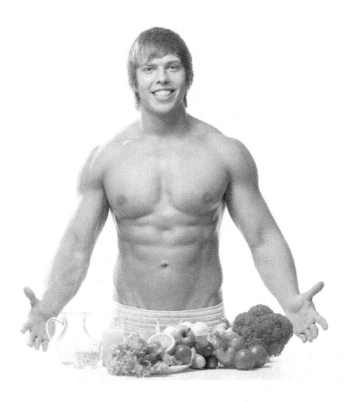

All types of vegetarianism have their own characteristics. Each of them with a reasonable approach brings great benefits to life. When you are faced with a choice of which type of vegetarianism to choose, you must clearly understand the reasons for your choice. Someone comes to vegetarianism because of health problems or a desire to maintain and improve health. Other people refuse meat products out of pity for animals. Someone decides to simply try for the sake of experience and remains on this path.

When choosing the type of nutrition, ask yourself a clear question: "Why do I need this?"

When you answer this question, it will be easier to understand which type of vegetarianism is closer to you.

A sharp transition to a strictly vegetarian diet almost always leads to protein starvation, as the body is accustomed to an excess of protein in meat products. Such stress can be harmful to the body.

When switching to a Lacto-ovo-vegetarianism or lacto-vegetarian diet, no negative consequences are observed.

Lacto-ovo-vegetarianism is the most liberal type of vegetarianism and provides the most favorable conditions for nutrition, in the best way combining health benefits and convenience in life.

Also lacto-ovo-vegetarianism does not violate your normal social life. This type of vegetarian food is extremely convenient - currently, it is difficult to find a restaurant whose menu is not suitable for lacto-ovo-vegetarians, and you do not need to refuse to meet friends in the restaurant. In almost every restaurant, a lacto-ovo-vegetarian will be able to choose different dishes and desserts to his taste that will not violate his diet.

Lacto-vegetarianism is very often a transitional style of nutrition, thanks to which people switch to a vegan (strictly vegetarian) lifestyle.

It is safe to say that a lacto-vegetarian diet is the most suitable type of vegetarian food for residents of modern cities from an economic, ethical and medical point of view.

In any case, you decide whether you will become a lacto-, ovo- or another vegetarian or vegan and what principles of nutrition you will follow.

High-Protein plant-based sources for Build Muscle

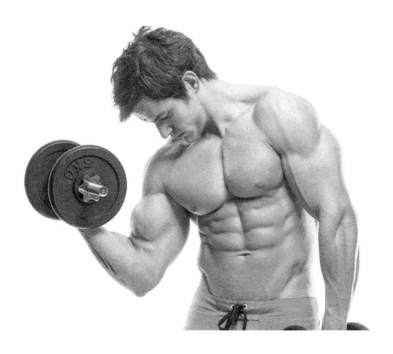

Protein intake is the main problem of many who want to switch to a vegan diet. Your decision to start a vegan diet means you have to be more watchful of the balance of nutrients in your diet.

We all know that nature is an excellent source of protein. So why not healthily build muscle without using meat products?

So, we provide all the necessary facts about the best sources of protein for a vegan diet.

So what are high protein plants?

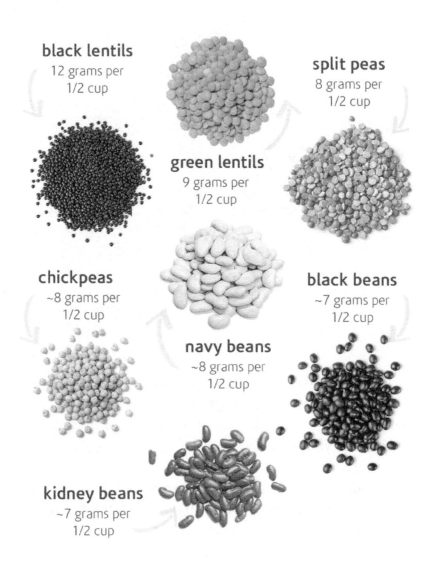

black lentils
12 grams per
1/2 cup

split peas
8 grams per
1/2 cup

green lentils
9 grams per
1/2 cup

chickpeas
~8 grams per
1/2 cup

black beans
~7 grams per
1/2 cup

navy beans
~8 grams per
1/2 cup

kidney beans
~7 grams per
1/2 cup

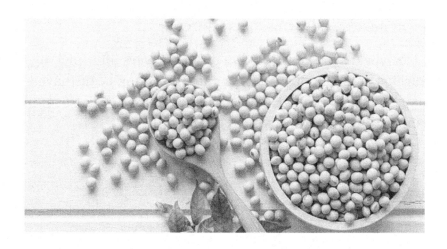

It would be remiss to not begin with everyone's favorite go-to protein plant. Popular with traditionally vegetarian populations in the East soya beans are a popular basic food for a large percentage of the population.

Soya beans always top the list, and it's no surprise

These are more like peas, as they grow in pods. In the western hemisphere they have gained popularity only this century, but soya products have been a valued protein source in the East for centuries.

China is the world's largest producer of soya beans in the world, supplying 80 percent of the basic soya products available. Soya beans are an intrinsic part of the traditional cuisine, taking on many elaborate forms. Cooked, made into pastes and purees, fermented and sauced.

Soya is a super food in the vegan world. It is quite high in protein content, and soya derived milk compares well to other plant milks in nutrients and texture.

Soybeans are processed in different ways after picking. The various methods of preparing and preserving beans have given us fermented, cooked, sauced and used as a base to countless concoctions including soy sauce and tofu.

Legumes: beans, pulses, lentils, chickpeas etc.

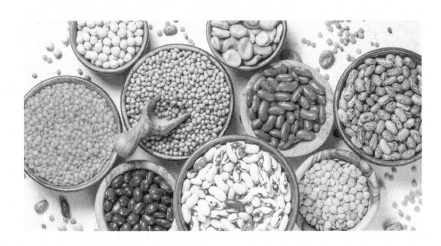

Beans, pulses, lentils, chickpeas are legumes. So are peas, beans, peanuts and anything that grows in a pod. Legumes are high in protein but not high in fat, so they are generally consumed as a healthy choice for meeting protein requirements as they can be consumed in large quantities without adding too many calories.

There are as many varieties of beans as there are colors of beans:
Black, white, red, green, brown and in between and many

varieties, the different colors indicating small variations in nutrients - black beans, white beans, cannellini beans, red kidney beans, speckled red beans, lima beans - and that is not even a list of half the beans available.

Here is a list of the protein levels of some common legumes per 100g:

- ➤ Soybeans - 34.9g
- ➤ Lentil - 24g
- ➤ Crushed peas – 23g
- ➤ Beans – 21g

Beans

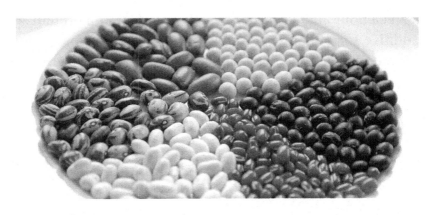

Beans are a popular vegan main source of protein, with the added benefit of slow digesting carbohydrates.

In the same category of high protein yield and low GI carbs you would also find pulses and lentils.

Pulses

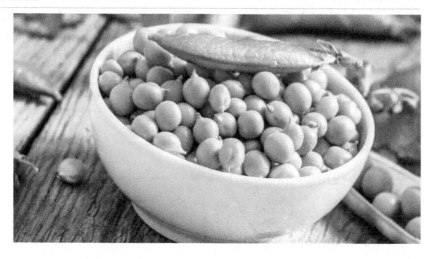

While not exactly lentils, pulses are different in their botanical classification and not in their protein content.

Pea flour and pea protein is very popular as a protein shake additive for athletes and bodybuilders, and anyone generally needing to increase their protein intake in an easily digestible form.

Lentils

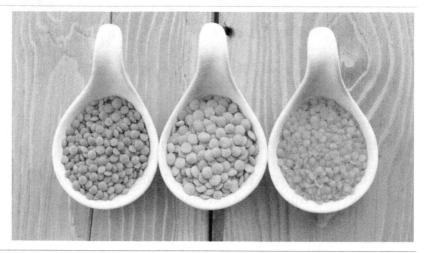

Lentils can be a great main course for lunch, or you can use it to make a vegetarian burger or meatballs.

Legumes and lentils can add protein to your meal without taking up too much space on your plate if you add them to your meal. This is a good way to increase your total protein intake per meal.

Chickpeas

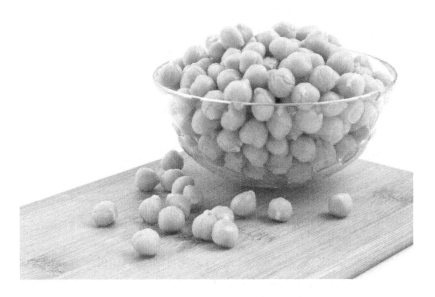

Chickpeas are high in protein, when cooked they contain around 14.5g protein per cup. Chickpeas can be eaten at any temperature and texture, and are highly versatile. Many traditional recipes that have been made for hundreds of years use these. They can be added to stews, boiled and pureed into hummus and dips, made into stir-fries and curries, or spiced and gently roasted in the oven.

Hummus made from chickpeas is a great spread, dip or protein-rich puree. It's made from pureed chickpeas and provides B vitamins and protein in the diet. Use it as a butter to add protein to your plate.

Nuts - peanuts, walnuts and almonds. Nut butters

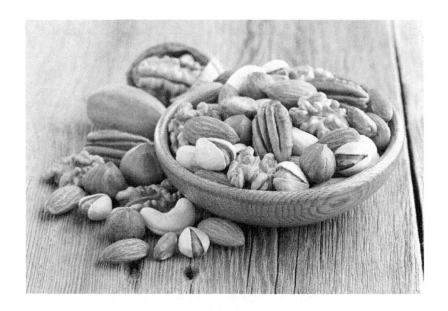

Vegetarians and vegans know the crunchy pleasure of indulging in larger quantities of nuts than people on a normal diet. Vegans can be a little less conscientious about avoiding fat. In fact vegans need to consume a variety of nuts. Certain combinations of nuts combine to form a complete protein.

Peanuts are protein-rich, stuffed full of healthy fats, and can be beneficial to your cardiac health. Made into butter, peanuts are rich in protein, with 8 g per tablespoon, and versatile. Use it as a sandwich spread, added to smoothies, sauces and desserts.

Almonds contain a large amount of vitamin E, which is necessary for the health of nails, skin, and eyes.

Walnuts are very good for brain health because of their protein profile.

Any nut can be turned into butter, and more and more vegans are already finding almond or macadamia oil on supermarket shelves. Eat toast for breakfast with almond oil, which contains healthy fats and essential proteins.

Here is a list of the protein levels of some common nuts per 100g:

- ➢ Peanuts - 26.3g

- ➢ Cashew nut - 20g

- ➢ Almond - 18.6g

- ➢ Hazelnut - 16.1g

- ➢ Walnut - 15.6g

- ➢ Pistachio - 10g

Grains and seeds

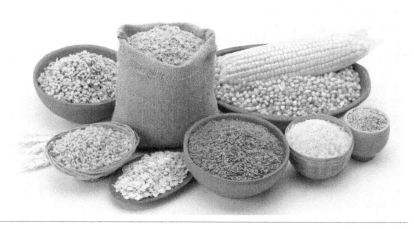

Seeds like quinoa are a complete protein. Quite impressive for this tiny seed. Other grains like millet, teff, amaranth, and sorghum also pack quite a large percentage of protein in a little package. They also make satisfying dense main ingredients to add to the main meal plate.

Seeds can be added to any meal or made into butter and pastes to add to the protein factor of a dish or side.

Grains are usually associated with carbohydrate load and something to be eaten in small amounts. They primarily add fiber to the diet. However, because of how versatile grains are, they can be added to any meal. As a food additive is easier to use grains as a filler, side or main, accounting for up to half of your protein intake for the meal.

Here is a list of the protein levels of some common grains per 100g:

> Oats - 26.3 g

> Quinoa - 24 g

> Wild Rice - 23.6 g

> Brown Rice - 14.7 g

> White Rice - 13.1 g

> Wheat groats - 11.3 g

> Oatmeal - 11 g

> Buckwheat - 10 g

> Semolina and corn - 10.3 g

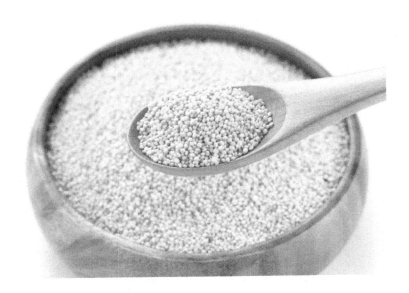

Quinoa is a seed (not a grain) with high fiber and surprisingly high protein content. Cooked quinoa contains 5 g of fiber and 8 g of protein per cup. The amino acids present in the seed form a complete protein, making it a unique plant food that is also rich in other nutrients, including magnesium, iron, and manganese.

While quinoa is known for its outstanding protein content, more recent health studies have shown it has some very real benefits. These are just some impressive nutrition facts about quinoa

Quinoa seeds are packed with flavonoids. They are high in protein content, dietary fiber, B vitamins, and essential trace minerals in larger amounts than any other grain. The black and red varieties contain betaxanthins and betacyanins. These phytonutrients provide antioxidant benefits from quinoa.

This is a very versatile and super-nutritious food. Versatile because you can prepare it as a salad, main or breakfast. It can be sprouted or cooked to varying textures - firm, or softer for breakfasts and dessert dishes.

Easy to digest, it's good for kids and grown-ups.

Flax, hemp, chia seed

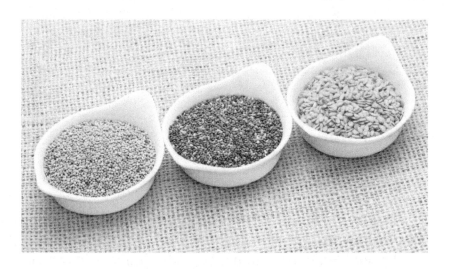

Flax seeds are high in Omegas and are a natural plant-derived and guilt-free way of getting your omega 3s and 6s.

Chia seeds are also high in protein and contain significant amounts of fiber. The tiny 'superfood' also has trace minerals Calcium, Manganese, Magnesium, and Phosphorous.

Hemp seeds are also a great protein source for people who get their protein from plants. Rich in fiber, protein and a range of fatty acids they also contain calcium, is a good source of plant-based iron, and magnesium.

Protein content in some seeds:

Nut/Seed (1/4 Cup)	Protein (g)
Chia Seed	12

Hemp Seed	10
Flax Seed	8
Sunflower Seed	8
Pumpkin Seed	7
Sesame Seed	7

Tofu, Edamame, Tempeh and meat substitutes

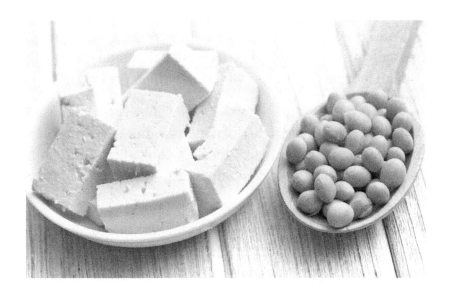

Tofu is a low-calorie food, though relatively high in protein and fat. Tofu contains many nutrients that make it a good protein source and meat substitute, mainly because of its chewy texture most of all. It is made by thickening soy milk and pressing into a solid block which can take on the texture of meat.

Edamame, Tofu, and Tempeh all come from soybeans. Soybeans are a whole protein. They, therefore, provide the body with all the essential amino acids needed.

Edamame are immature green soya beans, still in their pods. Edamame are rich in vitamin K, folate, and contain fiber. They need to be steamed or boiled to prepare them for use, and they can be used as a separate dish or added to your favorite salads and soups.

Tempeh, because it contains fermented beans, contains probiotics, B vitamins and minerals like magnesium and phosphorus.

Tofu is made from processed and pressed bean curd, pressed into solid blocks. Tempeh is made from lightly fermented ripe soybeans, which are then pressed into small blocks.

Tofu doesn't have a distinctive taste, but easily absorbs the flavor of the ingredients or sauce it's cooked in. Tempeh has a characteristic nutty flavor compared to the basic blandness of tofu.

Tempe and tofu can be used in various dishes to add protein and volume to the dish. All three products contain iron, calcium, and protein.

Sprouted and fermented plant foods.

Sprouted and Fermented Plant Foods are good sources of enzymes and probiotics.

Sprouted food is technically living food. The sprouting process begins the production of enzymes, many of which help to digest the fiber and protein in the plat. Fermented foods are also a wonderful source of living probiotics. The high concentration of living bacteria that is growing in the fermented food contains live cultures and enzymes, contributing to a healthy gut. This helps proper digestion of carbs and proteins.

Home-made sauerkraut, kimchi, lacto-fermented vegetables and drinks like kombucha add some fizz to your food and gut-healthy enzymes to your diet.

Mushrooms

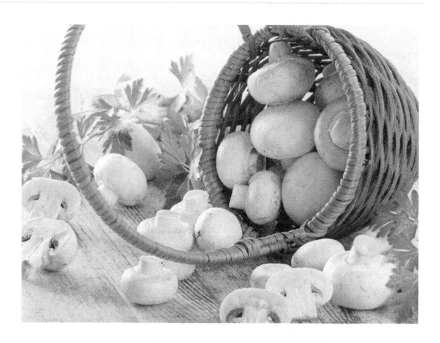

Mushrooms of all varieties should be present in large quantities in your plant diet. They are a good source of vitamin D if you do not drink milk.

Mushrooms in general and all edible species of mushrooms contain a large amount of vitamin D and iron.

Mushrooms are good for your health. For example, shiitake mushrooms have been used in medicine for hundreds of years.

Mycoproteins

Mycoprotein is protein grown from fungus and used widely as an alternative to a soy-based food product or as an alternative to meat products. Mycoprotein is a high fiber product and rich in essential amino acids.

Products with mycoprotein are used in cooked dishes as meat substitutes and are available in processed forms such as "chicken" nuggets.

Spirulina

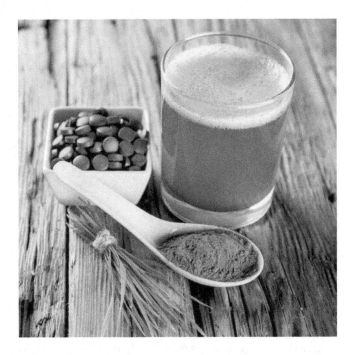

Spirulina is a blue-green alga harvested from the ocean. It is incredibly rich in nutrients, B vitamins (except vitamin B-12) and manganese. It contains around 8 g of protein per 2 tablespoons.

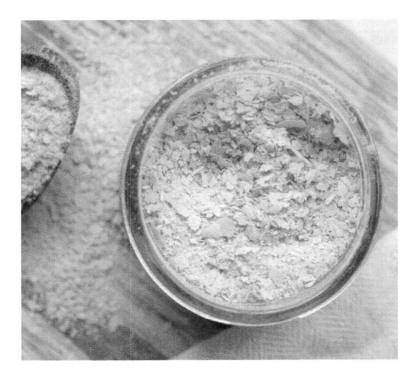

Nutritional yeast is a pungent odor powder. It contains B vitamins, especially B12 vitamins, which are mainly found in meat diets. The presence of many essential minerals makes it a great addition to a meatless diet.

Alternative Milk, Alternative Eggs, Alternative Cheese

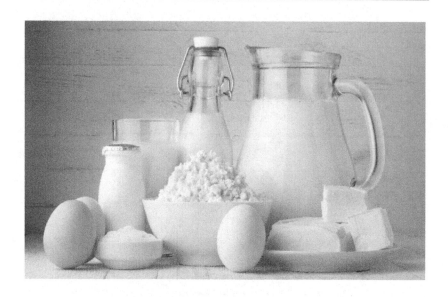

Alternative Milk

Lots of plant-based milk alternatives are as nutrients as typical dairy milk when consumed moderately. The list below shows the best alternatives for dairy milk:

Coconut Milk

This is a great duty-free alternative that can be easily gotten in grocery stores. It is manufactured by grinding coconut meat, and it is also a great source of nutrients like potassium, magnesium, and iron. Coconut milk also contains a medium-chain fatty acid called lauric acid, which is used by the body for energy. It is essential to know that full-fat coconut milk contains excess calories, yet it provides lots of health benefits; therefore you should consume little portions.

Goat Milk

Although goat milk is considered to be dairy but it is still an excellent alternative for those looking to stay away from cow products. Goat milk can be a bit different to digest, make you feel bloated, or affect your skin, yet it causes less digestive issues and inflammation than cow milk. Goat milk is endowed with adequate unsaturated fatty acids and also contain more medium-chain and short-chain fatty acids.

Almond Milk

This is a blend of water and finely ground almonds, which are a great alternative to dairy milk. It doesn't contain lactose, gluten or soy proteins, and it has anti-inflammatory properties. Unlike dairy milk, almond milk is more comfortable to digest, but almond milk is that it is often fortified with many additional nutrients and sweetened with added sugar. However, you should always go for organic, plain almond milk or you can decide to make it yourself.

Alternative Egg

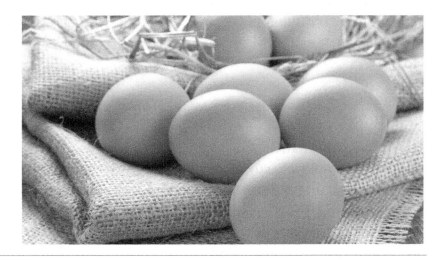

Turmeric

Turmeric gives a light yellow color when used in preparing egg-free dishes. It comes as a small root or in powdered form, and it is known to have anti-inflammatory properties. Turmeric can easily be purchased at grocery stores, and a little will provide an egg-like color to your food.

Apple Sauce

Making use of apple sauce is another way to substitute eggs in baked foods without adding eggs. Make use of a 1/4 cup of apple sauce (unsweetened) to replace a single egg. Apple sauce adds flavor and moisture to foods like cakes, bread, cookies, and muffins. However, they can be bought in stores or self-made by making use of fresh apples.

Black Salt (Kala namak)

Black salt is a volcanic salt that is used in Asian culinary art. As a result of it's concentrated sulfur content, it has a powerful flavor that tastes like eggs, making it a common ingredient used by vegans. It works brilliantly in vegan egg salads, tofu scrambles, vegan french toast, quiches, and frittatas. Black salt can be purchased online or at specialty stores.

Egg Substitute Powders

Various alternatives for egg substitute powders can be purchased in multiple stores. Vegan, gluten-free, and versatile, they usually contain flour or starch and a raising agent. They are also an excellent substitute for eggs when the volume is important. These powders won't add unwanted sweetness or flavor, and they can be used in cakes, muffins, cookies, and also as a building agent in vegan meatloaves or casseroles.

Tapioca Starch

Tapioca starch is used as a thickening or binding agent for condiments, sauces, and puddings. Make use of 1 tbsp of tapioca stare, grounded with 3 tbsp of water to substitute one egg. Tapioca starch is used to manufacture vegan mayonnaise, which is creamy and smooth, and it is considered to be a baking ingredient for most people.

Alternative Cheese

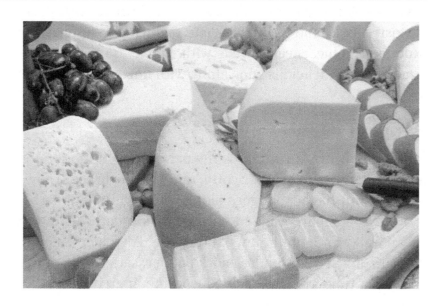

For Mozzarella — make use of daiya cheese:

The mouthwatering texture and stringiness of mozzarella can be difficult to prepare at home. However, this is why a dairy-free cheese such as 'Daiya' is recommended. Made with arrowroot, tapioca starch, potato protein isolate, and coconut oil, Daiya's shredded mozzarella (dairy-free) is the best option for making tacos, salads, pizzas, and quesadillas. Tapioca, which is gotten from root vegetable cassavas, can be used to represent a thickening agent in lots of food products, which include vegan cheese. It is easier to prepare and has the same healthy texture, but it stretches and melts.

For Blue Cheese — make use of herb and garlic cashew cheese:

If you prefer the spiciness of stilton or you prefer the nutty and sharp flavors of Gorgonzola, there are various kinds of blue cheese you can add to your dishes. The use of nutritional yeast, fresh minced dill, and garlic powder gives cashew cheese a tasty look and a great taste, which is comparable to Roquefort blue cheese. Dish with whole-grain crackers and crudites for a delicious wine along with faux-cheese spread.

For Ricotta Cheese — make use of almond cheese:

Almonds are known to be the perfect substitute for creamy cheeses like goat cheese, ricotta, and cream cheese. They have a subtle nut flavor that goes along with a variety of herbs and spices. To prepare almond cheese, soak 1 cup of almonds in clean water for a minimum of one hour. Then blend along with 1/3 cup of water, grounded black pepper, salt, and lemon juice. You can tune the flavor by including ingredients, such as minced garlic, dijon mustard, and natural yeast.

"Blacklist" foods for Vegan

What cannot be eaten by a Vegan?

Becoming a vegan seems simple enough. It would seem enough to avoid animal products - what could be easier? But this is not so. Many foods purchased in the store contain ingredients that either contain substances of animal origin, or, in one way or another, are associated with the exploitation of animals. In short, there are many foods that seem vegan, but vegans should avoid them.

Besides the commonly understood vegan no-nos, foods to say goodbye to forever include:

- all meat, poultry, and animal flesh;
- seafood;
- dairy products ;
- bee produced products like honey, beeswax, royal jelly, and pollen;
- food additives: some of them of animal origin, for example, E120, E322, E422, E 471, E542, E631, E901, and E904;
- dairy ingredients: whey, casein, and lactose are obtained only from dairy products;
- chips (may contain chicken fat or dairy ingredients such as casein, whey or animal-derived enzymes);
- white sugar, brown sugar, powdered sugar (it is better to replace them with maple syrup or agave nectar as a sweetener);

- some varieties of dark chocolate (contain animal products - whey, milk fat, milk powder, refined oil or skimmed milk powder);
- red products that owe their color to red pigments obtained from the bodies of cochineal females (insects). On the label, this ingredient is labeled cochineal, carmine acid, or carmine;
- margarine (may contain gelatin, casein (milk protein) and whey);
- pasta (some types of pasta, especially fresh ones, contain eggs);
- non-dairy cream (many varieties of such cream contain milk protein casein);
- Worcestershire sauce (spicy soy sauce with vinegar and spices): many varieties contain anchovies;
- gelatin (a product of the processing of connective tissue of animals);
- pepsin (the enzyme is present in the gastric juice of mammals, birds, reptiles and most fish);
- Vitamin D3 (most vitamin D3 is derived from fish oil or lanolin, which is present in sheep's wool);
- Omega-3 fatty acids (the source of most omega-3s is fish).

Even seemingly safe 'vitamins' can have animal origins or derivatives. As a vegan, you will get used to reading labels. In many countries, it is a legal requirement to declare specific ingredients, and this is definitely the case when animal products are involved.

Supplements to support the Vegan diet

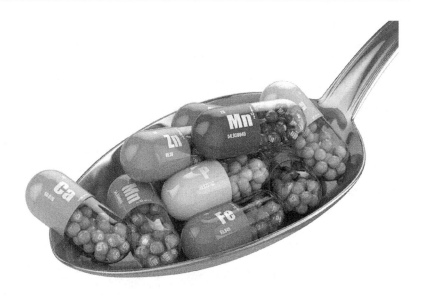

A vegan diet can be seen as a perfect blend of health and kindness to animal rights, the human body, and the environment. If you have definitely decided to follow a plant-based diet and avoid eating foods like meat, eggs, and dairy but choose to live on the consumption of legumes, vegetables, seeds, nuts, fruits and beans, then consider adding some additives to your diet to help keep you strong and healthy.

As already mentioned, a well-planned vegetarian diet can provide vegetarians with an adequate amount of all the necessary nutrients. However, the US Academy of Nutrition and Dietetics notes several important nutrients that vegetarians need to pay special attention to. Among them are iron, zinc, calcium and vitamin B12, vitamin D and omega-3 fatty acids.

Iron

Compared to non-vegetarians, vegetarians who refuse to eat meat may suffer from a lack of iron. It is emphasized that although studies have noted iron deficiency in vegetarians, iron deficiency anemia or a decrease in hemoglobin concentration have not been observed.

Vegetarians can reduce the risk of iron deficiency by eating fortified cereals and cereals, leafy green vegetables, tofu, lentils, seeds, nuts, and dried fruits.

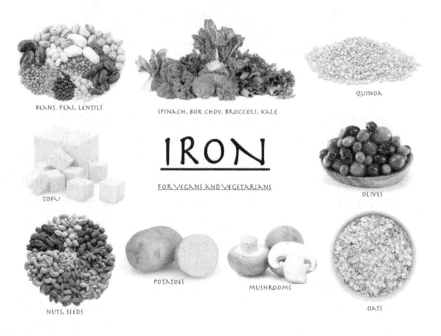

Zinc

As with iron, compared with omnivores, vegetarians absorb less zinc. Plants rich in this mineral, such as legumes, whole grains, nuts, and seeds, contain a lot of phytic acid, which violates the bioavailability (digestibility) of zinc. It is noted that especially vegans are in an increased risk zone. Taking zinc as a separate supplement may be warranted, especially for vegans.

Plant sources of zinc and zinc content:

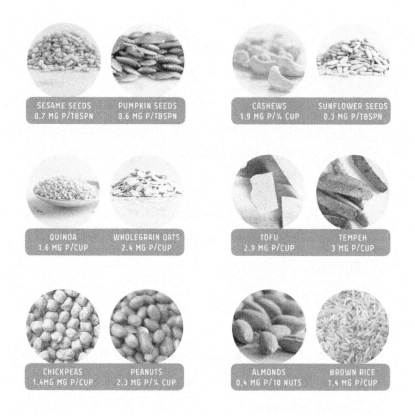

SESAME SEEDS 0.7 MG P/TBSPN — PUMPKIN SEEDS 0.6 MG P/TBSPN — CASHEWS 1.9 MG P/¼ CUP — SUNFLOWER SEEDS 0.3 MG P/TBSPN

QUINOA 1.6 MG P/CUP — WHOLEGRAIN OATS 2.4 MG P/CUP — TOFU 2.9 MG P/CUP — TEMPEH 3 MG P/CUP

CHICKPEAS 1.4MG MG P/CUP — PEANUTS 2.3 MG P/¼ CUP — ALMONDS 0.4 MG P/10 NUTS — BROWN RICE 1.4 MG P/CUP

Iodine

Iodine is known to be an important mineral for maintaining healthy metabolism and thyroid. Iodine deficiency can lead to slow metabolism, fatigue, weight gain, hypothyroidism, etc. It's best to consider sea vegetables when talking about iodine and a plant-based diet.

The list below shows the sources of iodine and a guide on how to achieve the recommended 150mcg daily (lactating and pregnant women have an increased recommended daily consumption which is about 270mcg for women lactating and 220mcg for pregnant women).

- Dulse Flakes (half teaspoon of this will give you the recommended 150mcg/day)
- Plant Proof Tip: Add the dulse flakes to your pepper/salt showered with these minerals. Therefore, there will be a hint of iodine whenever you season your food.
- Nori (to get the recommended 150mcg/day, ingest 1.5 sheets of standard Nori daily)
- Potatoes
- Wakame
- Cranberries
- Iodine sea salt (it is recommended to try and add the above food groups before including iodized salt as a source of iodine).

It is important to know that iodine is not a mineral you should go overboard with because when you eat too much quantity of iodine, you may develop hyperthyroidism or an overactive thyroid which can lead to weight loss, fatigue, heart palpitations, etc.

Calcium

Calcium is a very important mineral that helps maintain healthy teeth and strong bones. It is also crucial for muscle contractions, blood clotting and the healthy functioning of the nervous system. Getting the RDI of calcium can easily be achieved while on a vegan diet. For adults, it is recommended that 1000-1300mg of calcium should be consumed daily depending on gender and age (females and older people require more quality). The upper level is fixed at 2,500mg (1 year & older).

Below is a list of the top calcium-rich foods to help you decide on where to get your calcium from when you decide to follow a plant-based diet.

- Fortified plant milk (1 cup) — 300-500mg

- Kidney beans (1/2 cup) — 132mg

- Collards (1 cup) — 270mg

- Oats (1 cup cooked) — 84mg

- Hemp seeds (3 tbsp) — 20mg

- Tahini (2 tbsp) — 120mg

- Blackberries (1 cup) — 42mg

- Mustard greens (1 cup) — 160mg

- Kale (1 cup cooked) — 94mg

- Raspberries (1 cup) — 31 mg

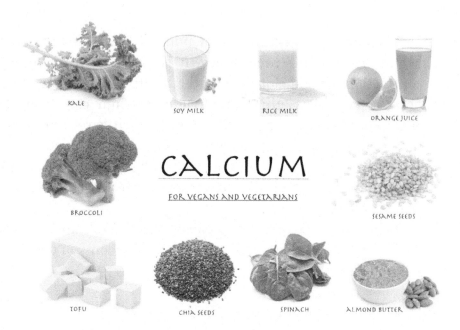

Vitamin D

Also known as the "Sunshine Vitamin" as a result of its ability to be synthesized by the body through the action of sunlight. Vitamin D is very important for increasing the absorption of calcium when required and promoting phosphorus absorption which promotions a healthy bone mineral density. The vitamin also plays a very crucial role in the brain, heart, immune system, muscles and thyroid. It also helps in regulating the production of insulin in the pancreas, which helps to fight against diabetes.

However, there are 2 main forms of vitamin D which are Vitamin D3 and Vitamin D2. Vitamin D2 is mostly artificially made by humans and combined with food substances via fortification. Vitamin D3, on the other hand, is synthesized from the sun into the human skin. It can also be found in few animal-based foods.

In winter months or when the exposure of the sun is limited, it is best to acquire vitamin D from a supplement. This is considered to be the most reliable and easiest way to avoid having a deficiency. Several studies indicate that 30-50mcg per day (100-200 IU per day) is effective for an average person to reduce the risk of dangerous diseases and develop a healthy vitamin D level.

However, the supplement dosage per serve can be expressed in IU (International unit) or mcg. 1 mcg of vitamin D3 is equivalent to 40IU, therefore if you are looking to get 50mcg of vitamin D daily, make use of a 2000IU vitamin D vegan supplement.

Vitamin B12

According to some estimates, 10 percent of vegetarians and 50 percent of vegans are deficient in vitamin B12. However, it is advisable to take about 2500 micrograms of vitamin B12 once a week or 500 micrograms per day, ideally in liquid or chewable form.

When the body lacks enough vitamin B12, it can lead to nerve damage, shortness of breath, fatigue, cardiovascular problems, inefficient transport of oxygen in the blood, and many other symptoms that are dangerous to health.

Vitamin B12 can be obtained mainly from animal products. Therefore, the addition of B12 following a vegan diet is not negotiable. This is because it is very important for the effective functioning of the body, and an adequate amount is difficult to obtain when consuming plants.

To cover the needs of this vitamin, vegans need to include enriched soy products in their diet - soy milk, tofu, and soy yogurt.

Omega 3 Fatty Acids

Omega 6's and omega 3's are to be fatty acids, and this implies that omega 6's and omega 3's are the only fats that the body system doesn't manufacture. Therefore, they have to be gotten from foods in our diet.

The average western diet consists of 20 times less omega 3's than omega 6's. This imbalanced ratio has very dangerous health consequences because a large consumption of omega 6's can lead to obesity, autoimmune diseases, cancer, and heart diseases. Basically, the omega 3/6 ratios protect the outer fatty layer of the cell in the body system.

One way of getting a long-chain of the recommended intake of omega 3's is by consuming adequate plant-based foods that have ALA. The NHMRC Dietary Guidelines recommend the consumption of 400mg/day of DHA/EPA omega-3 for optimal health. However, it is advisable to target a total of 8,0000mg of ALA daily because the body transforms at least 5 percent of ALA into DHA/EPA.

However, achieving the recommended dose is very visible, but can be difficult to maintain daily.

- 1 tablespoon of Ground Flaxseed gives 1600mg of ALA.

- 1 tablespoon of Hemp Seeds gives 850mg of ALA.

- 1 tablespoon of Chia Seeds gives 2000mg of ALA.

Therefore, you would require the consumption of 5 tablespoons of ground flaxseeds or 4 tablespoons of chia seeds daily, to make sure that your body gets adequate omega 3's.

Best vegan food sources of OMEGA 3 fatty acids:

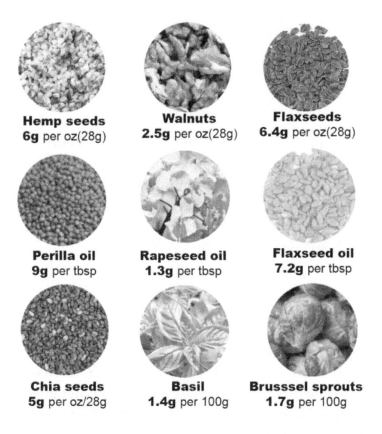

Hemp seeds
6g per oz(28g)

Walnuts
2.5g per oz(28g)

Flaxseeds
6.4g per oz(28g)

Perilla oil
9g per tbsp

Rapeseed oil
1.3g per tbsp

Flaxseed oil
7.2g per tbsp

Chia seeds
5g per oz/28g

Basil
1.4g per 100g

Brusssel sprouts
1.7g per 100g

How to start a Vegan diet?

Life hacks to go Vegan

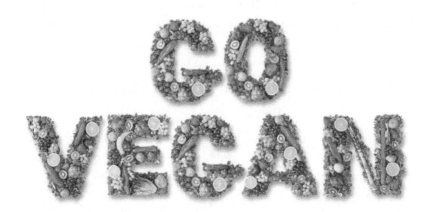

Thinking of becoming a vegan, but afraid of failure?

We will share with you simple and easy life hacks for how to become a vegan without harming your health. And these simple steps will help you to achieve your goal!

You do not need to follow them all, just take at least a couple of them and enjoy the process!

Transition slowly

Change too much at once might seem intimidating, but not when you transition slowly. If you push yourself too hard to do something which you're not prepared for, you might probably end up going back to your abandoned habits. However, it is best when you transition gradually. Begin by substituting two to three meals each week and when you get comfortable with it, you can then expand to add the remainder of your meals.

Replace animal products with vegan products gradually

Gradually remove meat and meat products from the menu, daily reducing their consumption. Do research on other plant-based dairy options and quietly add cheese or plant-based milk to your shopping list. However, you should also try to stop eating eggs. When you carry out this process a little, you will have the opportunity to adapt to a new dietary lifestyle, and it will be easier for you to truly devote yourself to this.

Find a vegan alternative to your favorite recipes

Do you like lasagna? Can't imagine life without a juicy burger? Has weekend ice cream become a tradition? Look for herbal recipes for your favorite dishes! Cook your favorite dishes with family recipes, turning them into vegetarian food. Now there is nothing impossible, the Internet offers a huge number of options for the same lasagna, burgers and ice cream without the use of animal products. Do not infringe on yourself, choose a replacement!

Eat your whole grains

Delete the notion that carbs are bad for your health because they are not. In fact, whole grains should become a primary source of energy for you. Not all carbs — or carb sources — are even. Heavily processed /refined carbohydrates are empty calories that lack fiber and nutrients. Whole grains (and all of the carbs they contain) are just fine. However, studies show that it is beneficial when a large portion of your diet comes from whole carbs. Foods such as rolled oats, brown rice, quinoa, farro, and barley will provide the adequate carbs needed.

Take snack whenever you're hungry

Most diets see snacking to be an enemy, but this won't be a problem if you snack on healthy foods. Grab something light whenever you're craving, you just have to make sure it's not junk.

Doing experiments in the kitchen

Use random plant foods in your kitchen and cook a brand new dish! Find vegan recipes, but add other ingredients and spices to them. Make the cooking process fun and exciting!

Try new food

Many people consider themselves choosy in food before switching to a plant-based diet. However, then they find food for themselves, which they could not even think of. Beans, tofu, different types of sweets from plants - such a meal for a meat lover seems tasteless. So try a new dish and let your taste buds decide for themselves what they like best.

Explore Tofu

To research? Yes! Tofu is a versatile product from which you can cook breakfasts, hot dishes, snacks, and even desserts.

It can be turned into similar ricotta, pudding, you can just season and fry or bake. Explore this product to turn it into something magical!

Cooking the legumes correctly

To avoid flatulence, prepare the legumes correctly. Soak them at least overnight and cook until cooked. You can also add asafoetida at the end of cooking, which helps the body digest these foods better.

Join communities on social networks

There are a billion vegan groups and communities on Facebook, Twitter, Instagram, and many other social networks. This is useful because you can find like-minded people and connect with other vegans. People publish recipes, tips, news, articles, and answers to popular questions. A huge variety of such groups will give you the opportunity to find a place that suits you best.

Find a vegan mentor

There are many organizations and services that offer mentor programs for a new type of food for you. You can write to him, and he will certainly give you advice and support. If you already feel like an expert in veganism, register and become a mentor yourself. You can become a distributor of a healthy lifestyle by helping someone else.

Read the labels

Learn to read labels of products, clothes, and cosmetics, look for warnings about possible allergic reactions. Packaging usually indicates that the product may contain traces of eggs and lactose. Some manufacturers put a vegetarian or vegan sign, but it is still important to read which ingredients are included. Read the labels carefully for "hidden" ingredients such as rennet, gelatin, etc.

Consult your doctor about nutritional supplements

Talk to your nutritionist or doctor to find out if you need nutritional supplements or special vitamins to make up for a lack of health-important elements.

Do not be afraid to waste time on the transition

The best transition is a slow transition. This applies to any nutrition system or diet. If you are determined to become a vegan, but now there are still animal products in your diet, do not give up on them suddenly. Discard animal products gradually, let the body get used to new healthy foods. Smooth transition avoids health problems and preserves your nervous system.

Vegetarianism and Bodybuilding

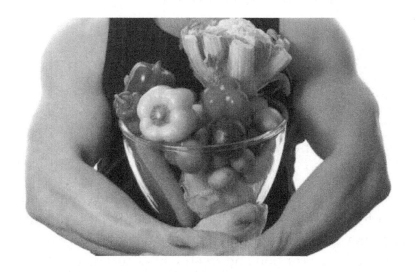

Do you often hear comments such as:
- Bodybuilder vegan? C'mon ... It can't be!
- Oh, are you a vegan? Where do you get protein from?
- Building muscle without meat? It's impossible!

If you're a vegan, you've probably heard these a million times.

So is it possible to follow a vegetarian way of life and do bodybuilding at the same time?

There is an opinion among people that it is impossible to pump muscle mass without eating meat. But, as professionals have proven, this is an achievable task.

Are vegetarianism and bodybuilding compatible?

A vegetarian diet gives the body no less energy than a meat diet. You just need to keep track of the variety of foods consumed daily to ensure the right set of nutrients.

Vegans don't necessarily build muscle slower than meat-eaters. There is more evidence to suggest that body type and personal protein metabolism play a much bigger role in how you develop stronger and larger muscles.

Opinion of official vegetarian and nutritional organizations about vegetarianism

American Dietetic Association

«Well-designed vegetarian diets, including vegan ones, are healthy and full, suitable for people of all ages, pregnant and lactating women, children, adolescents, athletes, and can also help in the prevention and treatment of certain diseases.»

Board member of the American College of Sports Medicine, Professor Tom Best, in his article for EAS also notes:

"Vegetarian athletes can satisfy their protein needs both predominantly and exclusively from plant sources, provided that these foods are consumed daily in a variety and calorie intake is sufficient to achieve their goals."

BNF - British Nutrition Foundation

«A balanced vegetarian or vegan diet can be complete, but more extreme diets, such as cheese-feeding, are often ineffective and do not provide a full range of essential micronutrients, making them entirely unacceptable for children. ...Studies of vegetarian and vegan children in the UK have shown that they develop and grow within normal limits.»

"A plant-based diet is now recognized not only as a complete diet but also as one that can reduce the risk of many chronic diseases.

The vegetarians' classic menu should consist only of useful products and should be diverse. It is essential to learn how to maintain a balance of nutrients and vitamins. You can diversify your menu if you start to pay attention not only to the usual and favorite products but also to those that have not yet dared to try. Another important rule of thumb is to eat more often and in small portions during the day and try different tastes because, in addition to biological processes, the interaction and combination of different tastes during the day helps circulation and processing of various emotions. I wish everyone good health, peace, and love. Nourish with health benefits.»

"Nutritionists of Canada"

«A properly planned vegan diet has many benefits, including reducing the risk of obesity, heart disease, high blood pressure, blood cholesterol levels, type 2 diabetes, and some cancers.»

How does veganism affect your muscles?

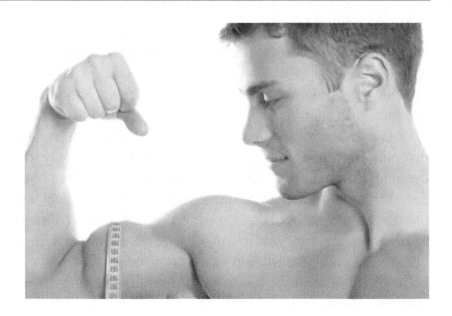

Vegan athletes and bodybuilders have special dietary needs. If you think about nutrition as being unique to an individual's needs, there is no one-size-fits-all. Similarly, there is no one-diet-fits-all. We all have specific dietary needs if we pay attention to our bodies and our eating. Vegans working out with the to rebuild their body, have to be extra vigilant of their protein intake and expenditure.

The amount of protein that you need to eat depends on your exact workout routine, the type of your body, how long you have not eaten meat, and other factors.

There are many unique eating plans for a vegan eating purely plant-based proteins.

In most cases, plant proteins need to be combined to form a complete protein, as you would find occurring naturally in animal sources.

It is worth noting that muscle-building would not be possible without particular vitamins and additives. These sports supplements are taken even by sportsmen for whom meat is a regular source of food and that do not eat chemical complexes.

There is a specially balanced diet for vegetarian athletes.

A balanced and proper diet is the key to good health and, if you want to gain muscle mass, it is the key to success. To do this, you need to include not only protein but also fats and carbohydrates on your menu.

From the right menu, the vegetarian can achieve the right amount of protein for muscle growth. Lacking components can be replenished with special sports additives. However, it should be remembered that muscles will not grow only due to excessive intake of protein. Fats are also necessary for proper muscle growth. And if there are no or not enough fats in the diet, this will also affect the appearance of the athlete, and their body will become flabby, their hair will fall out, and their muscle mass will become weak. Therefore, it is necessary to use vegetable oils, coconut milk, and, if vegetarian principles allow cow's milk

Scientists have proven that muscle building does not require as much protein as carbohydrates. But both play a significant role in this process. The protein itself needs to be eaten at a minimum of 1.6 grams per kilogram of weight.

Keep in mind that no expensive additives can replace a full meal. And, if there is a lack of carbohydrates in the diet, but a large amount of protein instead, the body will transform it into carbohydrates itself. Thus, the athlete will only harm his health.

The number of meals should be increased to six a day. These should be five main meals, and one before bedtime. With this approach, the muscles will continuously receive the necessary components, which means it will be much easier to build muscle. Not feeling hungry and at the same time, not overeating - this is the golden balance that any bodybuilder wants to achieve. If you do not follow this advice, the body will experience stress and store excess fat.

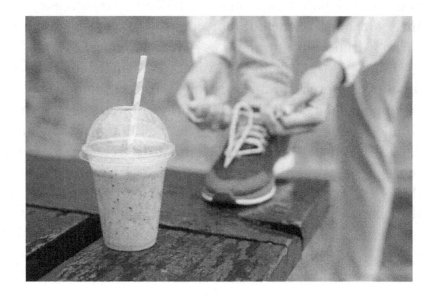

How to gain weight and build muscle on a Vegan diet?

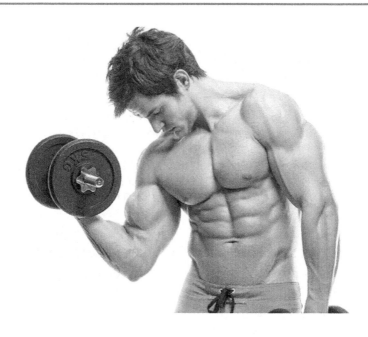

How much protein do athletes and bodybuilders need?

When you systematically exercise, your need for protein increases. To become stronger so that muscles can recover effectively, it is necessary to provide them with a sufficient amount of building material - protein.

The answer to this question is given by the authors of a study published in the International Journal of Sports Medicine:

- if you are engaged in power sports, then 1.4–1.8 g / kg per day;

- if you are fond of running or other endurance sports, then 1.2–1.4 g / kg per day.

(SOURCE OF INFORMATION: LEMON PW. DO ATHLETES NEED MORE DIETARY PROTEIN AND AMINO ACIDS? INT J SPORT NUTR. 1995 JUN;5 SUPPL:S39-61.)

The recommendations are consistent with the values published in the practice guide of the American College of Sports Medicine.

(SOURCE OF INFORMATION: RODRIGUEZ NR, DIMARCO NM, LANGLEY S; AMERICAN DIETETIC ASSOCIATION; DIETITIANS OF CANADA; AMERICAN COLLEGE OF SPORTS MEDICINE: NUTRITION AND ATHLETIC PERFORMANCE. POSITION OF THE AMERICAN DIETETIC ASSOCIATION, DIETITIANS OF CANADA, AND THE AMERICAN COLLEGE OF SPORTS MEDICINE: NUTRITION AND ATHLETIC PERFORMANCE. J AM DIET ASSOC. 2009 MAR;109(3):509-27.).

The International Society for Sports Nutrition published an article in its journal, which suggests consuming 1.4–2.0 g / kg of protein per day for most people involved in sports. Moreover, the authors of this article say that the daily norm of protein can be increased to 2.3–3.1 g / kg per day during a low-calorie period, and an increase in the daily amount of protein above 3 g / kg per day can contribute to weight loss!

(SOURCE OF INFORMATION: JÄGER R, KERKSICK CM, CAMPBELL BI, CRIBB PJ, WELLS SD, SKWIAT TM, PURPURA M, ZIEGENFUSS TN, FERRANDO AA, ARENT SM, SMITH-RYAN AE, STOUT JR, ARCIERO PJ, ORMSBEE MJ, TAYLOR LW, WILBORN CD, KALMAN DS, KREIDER RB, WILLOUGHBY DS, HOFFMAN JR, KRZYKOWSKI JL, ANTONIO J. INTERNATIONAL SOCIETY OF SPORTS NUTRITION POSITION STAND: PROTEIN AND EXERCISE. J INT SOC SPORTS NUTR. 2017 JUN 20;14:20.)

If you want to gain muscle mass, you need less protein than you think.

In general, a protein intake of 0.8–1.2 g / kg per day, as well as strength training and enough calories to maintain (or increase) weight, is the recipe for building muscle that you need. Why do we need such a seemingly not very large amount of protein per day for weight gain? The fact is that most visitors to gyms do not receive any additional benefits when consuming more than 1.7 g / kg of protein per day. Moreover, this amount can even decrease with the accumulation of experience, since with regular weight lifting, the body reacts better and there is muscle damage.

A study published in the Journal of Applied Physiology, in which 12 novice bodybuilders took part, evaluated the 4-week effect of consuming 2.6 or 1.35 g / kg of protein per day. The researchers did not find any differences in strength or muscle growth between the two groups.

(SOURCE OF INFORMATION: LEMON PW, TARNOPOLSKY MA, MACDOUGALL JD, ATKINSON SA. PROTEIN REQUIREMENTS AND MUSCLE MASS/STRENGTH CHANGES DURING INTENSIVE TRAINING IN NOVICE BODYBUILDERS. J APPL PHYSIOL (1985). 1992 AUG;73(2):767-75.)

However, it should be remembered that such studies evaluate the short-term effect, while the long-term impact is studied much less frequently.

Here's the rule for you: consume enough protein, but remember that "the more you eat, the better" does not work: you are more likely to consume extra unnecessary calories. Remember the nutritional balance.

The recommendations for the optimal amount of daily protein are different and may depend on various factors. To maintain sufficient flexibility in your diet, try to consume from 0.8 to 1.8 g / kg of protein per day, based on your goals: weight gain, reduction in fat percentage, maintaining lean body mass. In addition, it is crucial to consider your training load, training conditions, eating habits, food availability and several other factors. Perhaps you need extra protein to feel full, or, conversely, you need to reduce protein intake and calories in general.

Greek Yogurt	Lentils	Beans	Cottage Cheese
23 grams of protein per cup	4 grams of protein per 1/4 cup (cooked)	(chickpeas, black beans, etc.) 4 grams of protein per 1/4 cup	14 grams of protein per 1/2 cup

Hemp Seeds	Chia Seeds	Edamame	Green Peas
4 grams of protein per 1 tablespoon	3 grams of protein per 1 tablespoon	5 grams of protein per 1/4 cup (shelled)	8 grams of protein per cup

Quinoa	Peanut Butter	Almonds	Eggs
8 grams of protein per cup (cooked)	3.5 grams of protein per 1 tablespoon	3 grams per 1/2 ounce	6 grams of protein per large egg

The balanced ratio of proteins, fats, and carbohydrates for vegetarian bodybuilders

The entire set of macro- and microelements essential for our body to build muscle mass can be included in the menu of a "strict vegetarian" in sufficient quantities from plant foods. The following are the doses of macronutrients for vegetarian bodybuilders who want to build muscle, as well as recommendations for combining them.

Carbohydrates

Carbohydrates are considered to be the primary source of energy used during high-intensity activities. Studies indicate that including carbohydrates in the diet promotes performance and endurance. Based on per-calorie, the carbohydrate requirement for athletes is comparable to those for other people. Precise recommendations for athletes depend on activity type and weight.

Excess protein will not harm your health and body, but an excess of carbohydrates will immediately turn into undesirable fat, which will without doubt mask the defined abs you've worked hard for. Therefore, the best sources of sugars in the diet of bodybuilders are plant foods that have a low glycemic index and are rich in fiber. First of all, these are products such as rice, buckwheat, potatoes, dark flour pasta, and wholemeal bread.

Eating a large number of sweet fruits rich in fructose and generally eating sweet food, justifying it with the phrase "I now have a period of work for the mass, and I can afford to eat anything" is not recommended. You can never build powerful high-quality muscle mass if you do not tightly control the quantity and quality of carbohydrates in your diet. Usually, for muscle growth, it is enough to take in from 2 to 4 g of sugars per kilogram of body weight daily, dividing this dose into several servings, and eating these servings between 9.00 and 18.00. However, these figures are strictly individual and should be calculated based on personal data.

If you do not want unnecessary fat on your body, begin to calculate and control your daily dose of carbohydrates. Determine your exact daily dose of sugar. Twice a week in the morning, measure your waist circumference when inhaling and exhaling, as well as the volume of your arms, legs, chest. Keep a diary of your strength training, anthropometric data, and carbohydrate intake. Draw the right conclusions from the data. If there is no increase in strength and muscle volume, slightly increase your daily amount of carbohydrates.

If an increase in sugar does not contribute to an increase in results, but only increases the amount of fat on the stomach, reduce the amount of carbohydrates and start looking for your mistakes. Try to increase the amount of protein or healthy fats in your diet. Test your training system. Eliminate the possibility of overtraining, focus on basic exercises, while reducing the duration of the training and reducing the frequency of classes.

Proteins

Unlike carbohydrates, protein is minimally utilized for fuel. Its primary function is to maintain and build the body tissue. Plant-based protein sources are high, compared to animal sources, they have complex carbohydrates and fiber. The approved dietary allowance for the sedentary, lightly active, or average adult is 0.8 g for each kilogram of body weight daily. This tends not to be enough for the majority. In addition, protein requirements for athletes can vary from 1.2 to 1.7 g per kilogram of body weight daily.

Bodybuilders should take protein in an amount of 1.5 or even sometimes up to 5 g per 1 kg of your body weight. Usually, this is about 200-300 grams of protein per day. This protein should be complete, that is, its molecular structure should include all 8 basic proteins: valine, leucine, isoleucine, threonine, methionine, phenylalanine, tryptophan, lysine. The absence or insufficient amount of essential amino acids leads to growth retardation, weight loss, metabolic disorders, and in acute insufficiency - to death.

The principle of mutual complementation of proteins

The secret of vegans is the principle of complementarity (mutual complement) of vegetable proteins. This principle implies the intake of two or three different types of plant foods, each of which partially contains different essential amino acids. Amino acids that are not present in one source of vegetable protein can be obtained from another. In their training material entitled 'Proteins and Amino Acids in Sports', scientists from the EAS Academy, which specializes in nutrition for athletes, note that a combination of two or more plant-based protein sources makes it possible to produce a "complete" protein with essential amino acids. As a result of a combination of various sources of vegetable protein, we get the so-called complementary protein.

For example, breakfast consisting of lentil soup and wholemeal bread contains complementary amino acids that provide for the formation of a complete protein. Other examples are rice and beans, corn porridge or cornbread, and stewed beans.

A dish prepared from correctly selected plant components provides a complete set of complete proteins for muscle growth.

However, such food is rich in carbohydrates, which is good for gaining muscle mass, but is a negative factor during training.

Soy products and sports supplements in the form of soy protein can be considered a solution to problems with excess carbohydrates and a complementary diet, as soy protein is absolutely complete and contains all the essential amino acids.

It is worth emphasizing that there is no need for each meal to carefully combine plant sources of protein to achieve the complementarity of essential amino acids. The main goal is to consume a sufficient number of different sources of vegetable protein, which will complement each other, distributing their consumption throughout the day.

For example, if you eat low-methionine beans for breakfast, and then snack on almonds rich in this amino acid, you get the right amount of methionine.

Pay particular attention to sesame seeds, sunflowers seeds, and pumpkin seeds, as well as tofu. These foods are especially rich in Branched Chain Amino Acids (BCAAs), which help reduce muscle damage after training and are actively involved in protein synthesis.

COMPLETE VEGAN PROTEIN COMBINATIONS

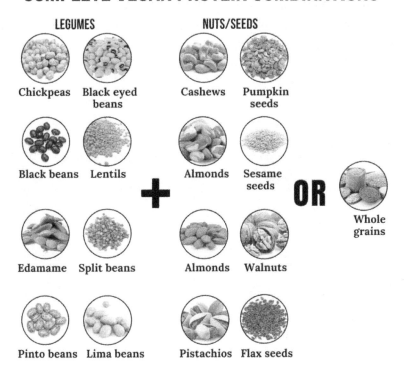

LEGUMES

Chickpeas   Black eyed beans

Black beans   Lentils

Edamame   Split beans

Pinto beans   Lima beans

NUTS/SEEDS

Cashews   Pumpkin seeds

Almonds   Sesame seeds

Almonds   Walnuts

Pistachios   Flax seeds

OR Whole grains

Fats

The traditional bodybuilding diet for gaining muscle mass suggests that 20% of the total calorie intake should be composed of fat. From the point of view of the biochemical composition, fat can be divided into three types: saturated, unsaturated and polyunsaturated.

Bodybuilders are advised to minimize the percentage of saturated fat in the diet by relying on unsaturated and polyunsaturated fats, as this can effectively solve problems with high cholesterol and excess subcutaneous fat.

A vegetarian can easily provide his body with the necessary amount of unsaturated fat, by including avocados, peanuts and cashews, olives and olive oil in the diet. Foods like almonds, walnuts, sunflower seeds, corn, and soybean oil are excellent sources of polyunsaturated fats.

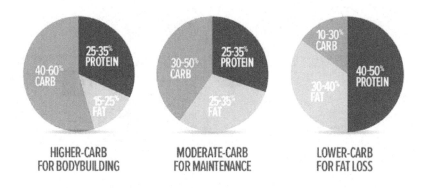

HIGHER-CARB
FOR BODYBUILDING

MODERATE-CARB
FOR MAINTENANCE

LOWER-CARB
FOR FAT LOSS

Useful tips for vegetarians bodybuilders

A vegan bodybuilder is a lifestyle

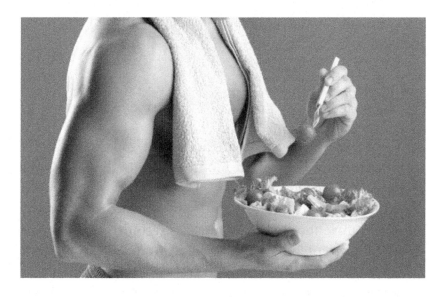

First, let's explain that the concept of nutrition for a vegan bodybuilder involves not only adequate protein intake, calorie control, and fat dosage. This is a certain system in which success depends literally on everything: the frequency of food intake, the total amount of proteins and dietary supplements are taken, the amount of fluid consumed, the combination of products and many other factors.

From how rationally the bodybuilder himself will be able to organize his diet - from the number of meals to the amount of water drunk - its result directly depends on a number of factors. Success, in this case, is a derivative of an integrated approach, and not just the influence of protein, as the followers of meat-eating believe.

Choose your type of nutrition

You must understand the difference between vegetarianism and veganism. Only you can decide what type of nutrition (lacto-, ovo-, lasto+ovo-, vegetarianism or strict veganism) is most suitable for you personally and corresponds to your lifestyle.

Eat real food

Forget about processed artificial food and gradually switch to natural: only from such food can the body draw strength and energy for itself.

Whole foods like nuts, legumes, vegetables, and seeds have enough nutrients that the muscles require and provide a steady supply of blood glucose and amino acid to muscles, unlike the nutritional dreck sold at the local supermarket.

Refuse fried foods in favor of cooked ones - this will greatly help your body and muscles.

Track your intake

The only possible way to find out if you are consuming foods adequately in the balanced proportions to develop the muscle is to record a fully detailed food diary and tally your macronutrients and calories.

Consult your trainer or nutritionist before making changes to your diet and trying to gain weight.

Calculate your daily calorie intake. When losing weight, people create a calorie deficit, that is, they burn more calories with their activity than they eat with food. To gain weight, you need to do the opposite: you need to get more calories with food than will be spent during the day. Ask your trainer for the correct calorie calculation just for you.

Consult your trainer or nutritionist before making changes to your diet and trying to gain weight.

Eat enough calories

The muscle is known to be a metabolically active tissue; therefore, you have to consume plenty of calories to keep it growing. If you aim to gain weight, consume around 20 calories for each pound of body weight daily. If you discover that 20 calories for each pound gathers fat and mass, come down to 15–17 calories. But this doesn't imply that you can consume pound pizzas. Quality is essential, therefore keep it clean.

Don't Shun Carbs

Half of the calories consumed per day should be carbohydrates - this is the "fuel" for the muscles.

To gain weight, you have to consume a lot of carbohydrates: about 3g for each pound of body weight. They contain glycogen to help with the intense lifting and calories needed for growth. Meals like brown rice, quinoa, oatmeal, and sweet potatoes are great options.

Don't shun fats

Fats are needed to deliver energy to muscles during training. The traditional bodybuilding diet for gaining muscle mass suggests that 20% of the total calorie intake should be composed of fat. Good sources of fats are olive oil, almonds, walnuts, avocados.

Pack in protein

Protein gives the amino acids which are used in developing the muscle. Opt for 1–1.6g of protein for each pound of body weight, or 180–270g a daily for a 180-pounder. We told you about the best plant protein options above. These products provide muscles with adequate amino acids for growth and recovery.

Mix various foods that contain protein: beans, nuts, lentils, chickpeas, peas, seitan (vegetable meat), greens, seeds, sesame seeds, soy milk, tofu, quinoa. Then your body will receive the full range of amino acids necessary for muscle growth.

Rise & Dine

When aiming to gain mass, consume 2 breakfasts. This will help you refill your liver glycogen and put a stop to the catabolism which chips away overnight, take in 2 scoops of whey protein, and a fast-digesting carb-like fresh fruit or smoothie after waking. After about 60 minutes, consume wholefoods breakfast that contains adequate protein—like beans, pulses, lentils, chickpeas, tofu, edamame, tempeh —and slower-burning carbs, like oatmeal.

Do not skip meals

Eat 5-6 times a day, in small portions. Your daily meal should consist of breakfast, lunch, dinner and two or three healthy snacks.

Make sure at least one portion of green salad per day is present in your diet - the amino acids contained in it will contribute to muscle growth.

Also, eat fruit for breakfast - this will not only give your body useful substances but also wake it up, stimulating it to act. After all, for an athlete starting the day right is the key to a successful day!

Drink plenty of water regularly

You need to drink a lot of water - at least 8-10 glasses a day. You can also get a good amount of calories with fluid. Use soft tofu, soaked nuts, seeds, and unrefined oils. Just add them to your smoothie!

Munch before bed

Before going to bed, consume some healthy fat and protein smoothie. As you sleep, proteins will slow catabolism by supplying a steady amount of amino acids About 40 minutes before you sleep, eat a cup of tempeh or tofu combined with 2tbsp of flaxseed oil or 2 ounces of seeds or nuts.

Mode of training and rest

To gain muscle mass, you need a good sleep and rest, because the muscles grow at this time, and not during training.

Add nutritional supplements if necessary

If you notice cramping in your legs during exercise or at night, then you are short of sodium and potassium. Try to increase the intake of these elements in the body - for example, nutritional supplements will help.

If you are troubled by sleep problems, add zinc and magnesium to your diet, which will help your body relax after exhausting workouts.

Pay special attention to foods that are rich in iron, zinc, calcium, vitamins D and B12, as well as omega-3 acids.

Plan ahead

Getting back from a workout session, tired and exhausted can tempt you to consume foods you shouldn't. But preparing enough protein-packed meals which can easily be microwaved will lead you to make healthy choices and gain the nutrients needed by your muscles. Make good use of your weekends to prepare big batches of hard-boiled eggs, chicken (if you are an ovo-vegetarian or have not entirely excluded animal products from your diet), rice, chili and stews, which can be frozen for the whole week.

Different body types. Vegan eating for your body type.

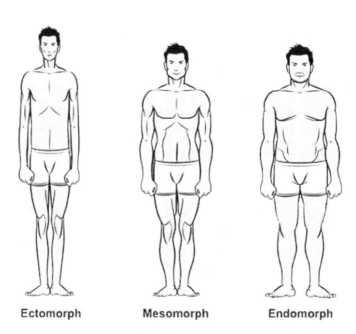

| Ectomorph | Mesomorph | Endomorph |

WHAT'S YOUR BODY TYPE?

Are all bodies suited or easily adapted to plant-based diets?

If you are someone who 'works out' and 'trains' at a gym, then you are familiar with the classification of body types and other body-builders well-known secrets. Bodies come in different shapes, sizes, and metabolic types.

Bodybuilders, athletes, and physical trainers of all kinds understand through intuition and study, that bodies are unique, but they seem to all fit into one of three body types. We take a brief look at the main body types and give a quick overview of each type's characteristics.

Classification of the physical body type is the most simple and obvious classification. Bodies can be divided into three main types.

Ectomorphs

An ectomorph is lean muscled and long boned, with slow-building muscles. They are generally slim and do not put on bulk easily. Ectomorphs need to be especially disciplined with regular workouts as their mass building is slow but steady.

Work with a trainer and consult a nutritionist to determine the optimal training regimen for building muscle. You must eat protein at every meal, so find ways to include protein as the main part of every meal.

This body type generally does better on a diet with a higher proportion of carbohydrates, with lower fat intake and moderate protein. The nutrient distribution for this body type must be:

55% carbs

25% protein

20% fat

Endomorphs

An endomorph belongs to the larger boned people group with high body fat as well. Men and women of this body type display a solidly built, almost pear-shaped lower half and they tend to store body fat easily.

These people typically do best on a higher fat and protein diet. This type should indulge in carbohydrate intake after exercise when it is metabolized better. A diet higher in fat and

protein, and lower in carbohydrates suits an endomorph best. The nutrient distribution for this body type must be:
40% fat
35% protein
25% carbs

Mesomorphs

The mesomorph body type is a solid, well-built, muscular type with a high metabolism and muscles that respond well weight training exercise, gaining muscle easily. They are not particularly prone to storing fat if they do not become too sedentary.

Mesomorphs have a medium-sized bone structure and athletic bodies carrying a more significant percentage of lean mass than the other body types. Mesomorphs are growth hormone and testosterone dominant.

The mesomorph typically does best on a balanced diet, mixing carbohydrates, proteins, and fats in a nutrient split of:
40% carbohydrate,
30% protein,
30% fat

Eating for your body type depending on your carbohydrate tolerance

As we become aware of how detrimental eating animal products can be on our bodies, we also become more tuned in to how different foods influence our metabolism and bodies.

One of the first things you should work out when you start exercising seriously to build muscle and mass is your carbohydrate tolerance and requirements

Your ability to handle carbohydrates improves significantly when you are physically active and it does not depend on your body type, body composition, or general physical condition. Thus, the best time to eat most of these starchy (or, ideally, less sweet) foods is when you are most active.

Various specific genetic and ethnic factors can influence how your body metabolizes sugars and the carbohydrates they break down into.

Depending on your body's carb tolerance and your body type, your fitness and bodybuilding strategy should be worked out to match.

Carbohydrate tolerance: High

If you are a very carb tolerant type, eating a greater percentage of carb-dense foods outside your workout times is suitable for you, This means eating more carbs throughout the day. You should ensure you get plenty of carbs around your workout for fuel and recovery. Remember that with an increase in carbohydrate intake, fat intake must necessarily decrease.

Carbohydrate tolerance: Moderate

If you know your tolerance for carbs is moderate, make sure you eat some carb-dense foods around your workout. If you have moderate carb needs, you should likely maintain a moderate intake of carb-dense foods outside your workout window. The rest of your meals would consist of less carb-dense foods and more lean proteins, vegetables, fruits, seeds and nuts.

Carbohydrate tolerance: Low

If your carbohydrate needs are low, your best option is to minimize carbs outside your workout window. This means eating mostly vegetables and low GI fruits, adding proteins and fats when you are not working out.

Sculpting your body means working with your body type and specific metabolism to achieve the shape you are working your body towards, especially if you know the type of fuel your body works best off.

Vegans, more than normal eaters who watch their protein intake less, understand that being aware of your body's reaction to food types can guide you to eating for your body by being aware of how you react to times and types of food. Some people love that comfortable feeling carbohydrates can wrap you in, and others prefer the mental sharpness a high protein/fat diet can give you. As you keep exercising and tailoring your carb, protein and fat intake, your body will change, along with your understanding of how you should eat for your body type.

VEGAN COOKBOOK with High-protein Recipes for Healthy Weight Gain and Build Muscle

High Protein Breakfast

Breakfast Burritos

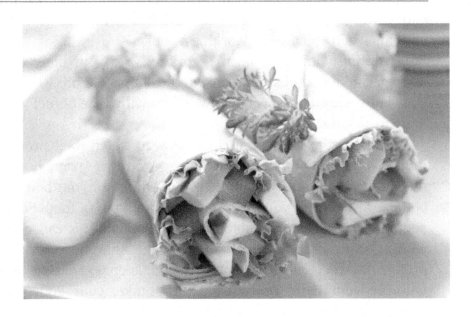

Total Time: 20 minutes | Servings: 4

INGREDIENTS:

2 (15 oz) cans black beans, drained and rinsed
½ cup of water
4 whole-wheat tortillas
8 leaves romaine lettuce
2 tomatoes, sliced
2 avocados, peeled, pitted, and sliced
1 ½ cups salsa

Seasonings:
1 tbsp garlic powder
1 tbsp onion powder
1 tbsp chili powder
1 tsp dried cumin
1 tsp dried oregano

Nutrition Facts		
Amount per		
1 serving (15 oz)		427 g
Calories 371	From Fat	170
		% Daily Value*
Total Fat 20g		31%
Saturated Fat 4.4g		22%
Trans Fat 0g		
Cholesterol 0mg		0%
Sodium 969mg		40%
Total Carbohydrates 45g		15%
Dietary Fiber 17g		67%
Sugars 7g		
Protein 10g		20%
Vitamin A 36% • **Vitamin C** 29%		
Calcium 22% • **Iron** 25%		
* Percent Daily Values are based on 2000 calorie diet. Your Daily Values may be higher or lower depending on your calorie needs.		

COOKING INSTRUCTIONS:

1. In a medium-sized pot, add the beans, water, and seasonings. Allow boiling over medium heat and then simmer for 10 minutes. Drain the beans after.

2. Onto the whole wheat tortillas, add one or two leaves of romaine lettuce, tomatoes, and avocado.

3. Add the black beans on top and then, the salsa.

4. Serve the burritos immediately.

Banana Pancakes

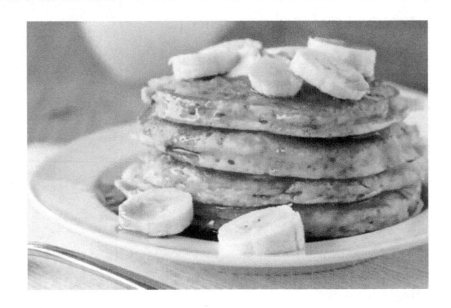

Total Time: 30 minutes | Servings: 4

INGREDIENTS:

2 cups rolled oats

1 tsp protein collagen powder

2 ripe bananas

1 cup unsweetened plant milk

2 tbsp olive oil

Toppings:

Chopped dates

Unsweetened fruit jam to taste

Nutrition Facts		
Amount per		
1 serving (4.3 oz)		121 g
Calories 232	**From Fat**	107
		% Daily Value*
Total Fat 12.3g		19%
Saturated Fat 2.7g		14%
Trans Fat 0g		
Cholesterol 6mg		2%
Sodium 31mg		1%
Total Carbohydrates 38g		13%
Dietary Fiber 8g		31%
Sugars 6g		
Protein 11g		21%
Vitamin A 3% • Vitamin C		1%
Calcium 10% • Iron		15%
* Percent Daily Values are based on 2000 calorie diet. Your Daily Values may be higher or lower depending on your calorie needs.		

COOKING INSTRUCTIONS:

1. In a blender, add the oats, protein powder, bananas, plant milk, and process on high speed until smooth, 2 minutes. If the batter is too thick, thin with some more plant milk.

2. Heat a ¼ of the olive oil in a medium skillet and add ¼ cup of batter. Cook until the edges slightly crisp and bubbles form on the surface. Flip and cook on the other side for 2 more minutes.

3. Plate and repeat the cooking process with the remaining butter and olive oil in the same proportions.

4. Top the pancakes with some jam and dates, and serve immediately.

Tofu Potatoes O'Brien

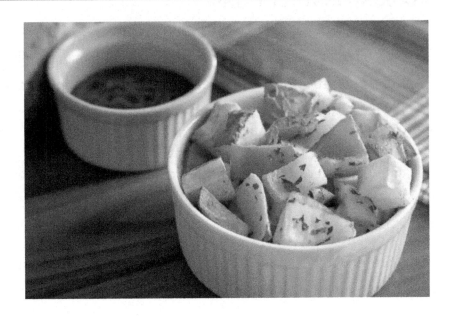

Total Time: 40 minutes | Servings: 4

INGREDIENTS:

2 tbsp vegetable oil
1 (14 oz) extra-firm tofu, pressed and cubed
4 large red potatoes, medium diced
1 small onion, medium diced
3 bell peppers (any color), medium diced
¼ cup of water
1 tsp sweet paprika
1 tsp garlic powder
1 tsp dried oregano
1 tsp dried thyme
Salt and black pepper to taste

Nutrition Facts		
Amount per		
1 serving (16 oz)		455 g
Calories 348	From Fat	66
		% Daily Value*
Total Fat 7.5g		12%
Saturated Fat 1.2g		6%
Trans Fat 0g		
Cholesterol 0mg		0%
Sodium 71mg		3%
Total Carbohydrates 66g		22%
Dietary Fiber 8g		30%
Sugars 8g		
Protein 8g		17%
Vitamin A 17% • Vitamin C 238%		
Calcium 6% • Iron		20%
* Percent Daily Values are based on 2000 calorie diet. Your Daily Values may be higher or lower depending on your calorie needs.		

COOKING INSTRUCTIONS:

1. In a large skillet with a lid, heat the vegetable oil over medium heat.

2. Sauté the tofu and potatoes until browned, 7 minutes.

3. Add the onion and bell peppers; continue to cooking for 3 minutes.

4. Stir in the spices and cook for a minute.

5. Pour the water into the skillet and cover with the lid. Reduce the heat to low and simmer for 5 minutes.

6. When ready, open the pot and adjust the taste with salt and black pepper.

7. Dish the food and serve warm.

Raspberry PB&J Overnight Oats

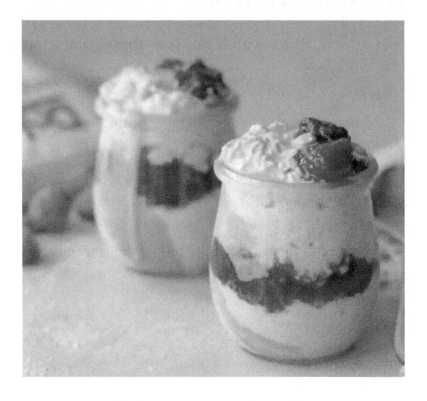

Total Time: 10 minutes | Servings: 4

INGREDIENTS:

4 large mason jars
2 cups rolled oats
½ cup peanut butter
½ cup raspberry jam
4 cups unsweetened plant milk
Sliced raspberries for topping

Nutrition Facts		
Amount per		
1 serving (12.7 oz)		360 g
Calories 386	From Fat	152
		% Daily Value⁴
Total Fat 17.1g		26%
Saturated Fat 6.2g		31%
Trans Fat 0g		
Cholesterol 24mg		8%
Sodium 589mg		25%
Total Carbohydrates 58g		19%
Dietary Fiber 9g		36%
Sugars 26g		
Protein 18g		37%
Vitamin A 8% • Vitamin C 5%		
Calcium 32% • Iron 17%		
* Percent Daily Values are based on 2000 calorie diet. Your Daily Values may be higher or lower depending on your calorie needs.		

COOKING INSTRUCTIONS:

1. Open the lids of the mason jars and pour in the ingredients in this order: ¼ cup rolled oats, 1 tbsp peanut butter, 1 tbsp raspberry jam, and ¼ cup rolled oats, 1 tbsp peanut butter, and 1 tbsp raspberry jam.

2. Add 1 cup of plant milk to each jar, cover with their lids, and then refrigerate overnight.

3. The next morning, remove the jars, open the lid, add the raspberries, and serve the oats cold.

Avocado Sandwich

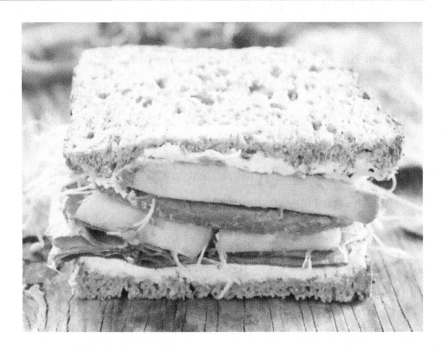

Total Time: 10 minutes | Servings: 2

INGREDIENTS:

8 whole-wheat bread slices

½ oz. vegan butter

2 oz. little gem lettuce, cleaned and patted dry

1 oz. tofu cheese, sliced

1 avocado, pitted, peeled, and sliced

1 small cucumber, sliced into 4 rings

Freshly chopped parsley to garnish

Nutrition Facts

Amount per
1 serving (7.8 oz)   220 g

Calories 473	From Fat 128
	% Daily Value*
Total Fat 15.2g	23%
Saturated Fat 3.6g	18%
Trans Fat 0.1g	
Cholesterol 8mg	3%
Sodium 606mg	25%
Total Carbohydrates 77g	26%
Dietary Fiber 14g	55%
Sugars 2g	
Protein 15g	31%
Vitamin A 30% • Vitamin C 42%	
Calcium 8% • Iron 31%	

* Percent Daily Values are based on 2000
calorie diet. Your Daily Values may be
higher or lower depending on your
calorie needs.

COOKING INSTRUCTIONS:

1. Arrange the 4 bread slices on a flat surface and smear the vegan butter on one end each.

2. Place a lettuce leaf on each and arrange some tofu cheese on top. Top with the avocado and cucumber slices.

3. Garnish the sandwiches with a little parsley, cover with the remaining bread slices, and serve immediately.

Mexican Tofu Scramble

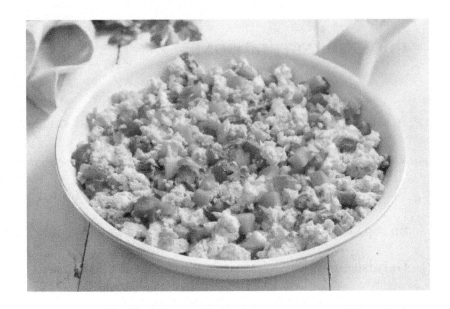

Total Time: 46 minutes | Servings: 4

INGREDIENTS:

8 oz water-packed extra firm tofu

2 tbsp vegan butter, for frying

1 green bell pepper, seeded and finely chopped

1 tomato, finely chopped

2 tbsp chopped fresh green onions to garnish

Salt and black pepper to taste

1 tsp Mexican-style chili powder

3 oz. grated vegan Parmesan cheese

Nutrition Facts

Amount per
1 serving (5 oz)   143 g

Calories 209	From Fat 133
	% Daily Value*
Total Fat 15.2g	23%
Saturated Fat 7.3g	36%
Trans Fat 0.4g	
Cholesterol 34mg	11%
Sodium 468mg	20%
Total Carbohydrates 8g	3%
Dietary Fiber 1g	4%
Sugars 2g	
Protein 13g	25%

Vitamin A 23% • Vitamin C 101%
Calcium 29% • Iron 9%

* Percent Daily Values are based on 2000 calorie diet. Your Daily Values may be higher or lower depending on your calorie needs.

COOKING INSTRUCTIONS:

1. Place the tofu in between two parchment papers to drain liquid for 30 minutes.

2. After 30 minutes, melt the vegan butter in a large non-stick skillet until no longer foaming.

3. Crumble the tofu into the skillet and fry with occasional stirring until golden brown, 4 to 6 minutes. Make sure not to break the tofu into tiny pieces. The goal is to have those resembling scrambled eggs.

4. Stir in the bell pepper, tomato, green onions, and cook until the vegetables soften 4 minutes. Season with salt, black pepper, chili powder, and stir in the cheese until well-combined and beginning to melt, 2 minutes.

5. Dish the food and serve warm.

Coconut French Toasts

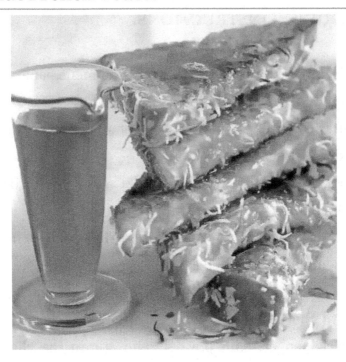

Total Time: 16 minutes | Servings: 2

INGREDIENTS:
For the glass dish bread:
2 tbsp. flaxseed meal + 6 tbsp water

1 tsp vegan butter

2 tbsp plain flour

2 tbsp almond flour

1½ tsp baking powder

1 tsp nutritional yeast

A pinch salt

2 tbsp coconut cream

For the toast's batter
2 tbsp. flaxseed meal + 6 tbsp water

Nutrition Facts		
Amount per		
1 serving (1.4 oz)		40 g
Calories 142	From Fat	88
	% Daily Value*	
Total Fat 10.2g		16%
Saturated Fat 6.8g		34%
Trans Fat 0.3g		
Cholesterol 18mg		6%
Sodium 114mg		5%
Total Carbohydrates 10g		3%
Dietary Fiber 1g		3%
Sugars 0g		
Protein 4g		8%
Vitamin A 5% • Vitamin C		1%
Calcium 11% • Iron		6%
* Percent Daily Values are based on 2000 calorie diet. Your Daily Values may be higher or lower depending on your calorie needs.		

2 tbsp coconut milk whipping cream
1 tsp almond extract
½ tsp cinnamon powder + extra for
garnishing
1 pinch salt
2 tbsp vegan butter

COOKING INSTRUCTIONS:
1. For the flax egg, whisk both quantities of flaxseed powder and water in two separate bowls and allow soaking for 5 minutes.

For the glass dish bread
2. Grease a glass dish (for the microwave) with the vegan butter.
3. In another bowl, combine the plain flour, almond flour, baking powder, nutritional yeast, and salt.
4. When the flaxseed egg is ready, whisk one portion with the coconut whipping cream and mix into the dry ingredients until smooth.
5. Pour the dough into the glass dish and microwave for 2 minutes or until the middle part of the bread is set.
6. Remove the ball, slice the bread and return to the glass dish.

For the toast
7. Whisk the remaining flax egg with the coconut whipping cream, almond milk, cinnamon powder, and salt until well combined.
8. Pour the mixture over the bread slices and leave to soak. Turn the bread a few times to soak in as much of the batter.
9. Melt the vegan butter in a frying pan and toast the bread slices on both sides.
10. Place the bread on a plate, garnish with some cinnamon, and serve warm.

Blueberry Chia Pudding

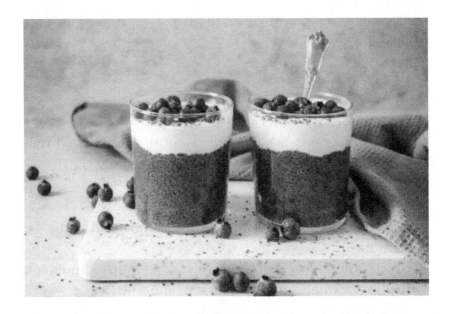

Total Time: 4 hours 3 minutes | Servings: 2

INGREDIENTS:

¾ cup of coconut milk

½ tsp vanilla extract

½ cup blueberries

2 tbsp. chia seeds

Chopped walnuts to garnish

Nutrition Facts

Amount per
1 serving (3.3 oz)   93 g

Calories 307	From Fat 250

	% Daily Value*
Total Fat 29.9g	46%
Saturated Fat 11.3g	57%
Trans Fat	
Cholesterol 0mg	0%
Sodium 8mg	0%
Total Carbohydrates 9g	3%
Dietary Fiber 3g	14%
Sugars 4g	
Protein 6g	11%

Vitamin A 0%	Vitamin C 6%
Calcium 4%	Iron 9%

* Percent Daily Values are based on 2000
calorie diet. Your Daily Values may be
higher or lower depending on your
calorie needs.

COOKING INSTRUCTIONS:

1. In a blender, combine the coconut milk, vanilla extract, and half of the blueberries. A process on high speed until smooth.

2. Open the blender and stir in the chia seeds.

3. Divide the mixture into two breakfast jars, cover, and refrigerate for 4 hours to allow the mixture to gel.

4. Garnish the pudding with the remaining blueberries and walnuts. Serve immediately.

Coconut Milk Coffee

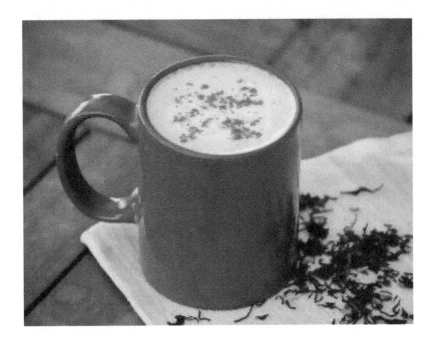

Total Time: 3 minutes | Servings: 2

INGREDIENTS:

2 ½ tsp ground coffee beans

1 cup of water

¼ cup of coconut milk

2 tbsp unsalted vegan butter

Nutrition Facts		
Amount per		
1 serving (2.9 oz)		81 g
Calories 69	From Fat	65
		% Daily Value*
Total Fat 7.4g		11%
Saturated Fat 5.6g		28%
Trans Fat		
Cholesterol 7mg		2%
Sodium 6mg		0%
Total Carbohydrates 1g		0%
Dietary Fiber 0g		1%
Sugars 1g		
Protein 1g		1%
Vitamin A 2% • Vitamin C		1%
Calcium 1% • Iron		2%
* Percent Daily Values are based on 2000 calorie diet. Your Daily Values may be higher or lower depending on your calorie needs.		

COOKING INSTRUCTIONS:

1. Using a coffee maker, brew one cup of coffee with the ground coffee beans and water.

2. Pour the coffee into a blender, add the coconut milk, vegan butter, and blend until frothy and smooth.

3. Pour the drink into two teacups and serve immediately.

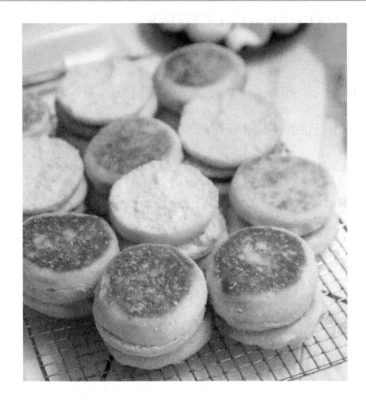

Total Time: 20 minutes | Servings: 4

INGREDIENTS:

2 tbsp flax seed powder + 6 tbsp water

2 tbsp plain flour

1 tsp nutritional yeast

½ tsp baking powder

1 scoop protein collagen powder

1 pinch salt

3 tbsp vegan butter

Nutrition Facts

Amount per
1 serving (1.1 oz)   30 g

Calories 119	From Fat	83
		% Daily Value*
Total Fat 9.4g		15%
Saturated Fat 5.5g		28%
Trans Fat 0.3g		
Cholesterol 24mg		8%
Sodium 129mg		5%
Total Carbohydrates 5g		2%
Dietary Fiber 0g		1%
Sugars 0g		
Protein 4g		8%

Vitamin A 10% • Vitamin C 4%
Calcium 11% • Iron 6%

* Percent Daily Values are based on 2000
calorie diet. Your Daily Values may be
higher or lower depending on your
calorie needs

COOKING INSTRUCTIONS:

1. In a small bowl, mix the flax seed powder with water and allow soaking for 5 minutes.

2. In another bowl, combine the flour, nutritional yeast, baking powder, protein powder, and salt. Pour in the flax egg, whisk well and allow the batter to sit for 5 minutes or until set.

3. Working in batches, melt the vegan butter in a frying pan over medium heat and add the mixture in four dollops. Fry until golden brown on one side, flip the bread with a spatula and fry further until golden brown.

4. Plate the muffins and serve with some vegan butter and tea.

Salads

White Bean & Tomato Salad

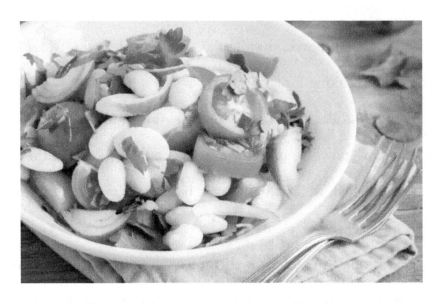

Total Time: 15 minutes | Servings: 4

INGREDIENTS:

For the dressing:

3 tbsp freshly squeezed lemon juice

¼ cup olive oil

1 garlic clove, minced

¼ tsp salt

1/8 tsp black pepper

For the salad:

2 (15 oz) cans white beans, drained
and rinsed

Nutrition Facts		
Amount per 1 serving (5 oz)		141 g
Calories 169	From Fat	12
		% Daily Value*
Total Fat 1.3g		2%
Saturated Fat 0.2g		1%
Trans Fat 0g		
Cholesterol 0mg		0%
Sodium 11mg		0%
Total Carbohydrates 30g		10%
Dietary Fiber 7g		29%
Sugars 2g		
Protein 11g		22%
Vitamin A 13% • Vitamin C		26%
Calcium 11% • Iron		25%
* Percent Daily Values are based on 2000 calorie diet. Your Daily Values may be higher or lower depending on your calorie needs.		

2 cups cherry tomatoes, quartered

½ small red onion, sliced

1 garlic clove, minced

½ cup chopped fresh parsley

COOKING INSTRUCTIONS:

1. Mix the dressing's ingredients in a large bowl until well-combined and add the white beans, garlic, tomatoes, onion, and parsley.

2. Coat the salad with the dressing.

3. Serve immediately.

Berry Salad with Arugula

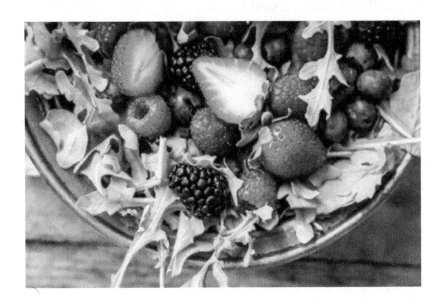

Time: 10 minutes | Servings: 4

INGREDIENTS:

For the dressing:

1 ½ cups fresh raspberry

¼ cup red wine vinegar

1 tsp Dijon mustard

1/8 tsp black pepper

½ cup olive oil

1 tbsp. spirinula

1 small shallot, diced

For the salad:

Nutrition Facts		
Amount per		
1 serving (9.6 oz)		272 g
Calories 362	From Fat	276
		% Daily Value*
Total Fat 31.8g		49%
Saturated Fat 8.9g		45%
Trans Fat 0g		
Cholesterol 33mg		11%
Sodium 541mg		23%
Total Carbohydrates 15g		5%
Dietary Fiber 6g		24%
Sugars 7g		
Protein 8g		16%
Vitamin A 32% • Vitamin C		69%
Calcium 24% • Iron		12%
*Percent Daily Values are based on 2000 calorie diet. Your Daily Values may be higher or lower depending on your calorie needs.		

6 cups arugula

½ cup blueberries

1 cup strawberries, halved

½ cup raspberries

1/3 cup red onion, thinly sliced

1/3 cup goat cheese, crumbled

¼ cup walnuts, roughly chopped

COOKING INSTRUCTIONS:

1. Add all the dressings ingredients into a food processor and blend until smooth. Set aside.

2. Spread the arugula in the bottom of a wide salad bowl and top with the remaining ingredients.

3. Drizzle the dressing on top, toss well, and enjoy immediately.

Grilled Tempeh and Chickpea Salad

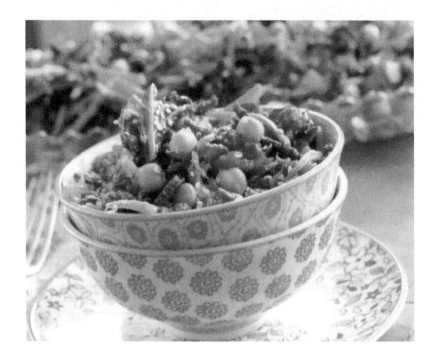

Time: 5 minutes | Servings: 4

INGREDIENTS:

4 tempeh fillets, grilled and chopped
2 (15 oz) cans chickpeas, drained and rinsed
1 tbsp drained capers
1 red onion, thinly sliced
2 tbsp olive oil
1 tbsp red wine vinegar
A pinch salt
1/8 tsp black pepper

Nutrition Facts		
Amount per		
1 serving (3.4 oz)		96 g
Calories 270	From Fat	240
		% Daily Value*
Total Fat 27.2g		42%
Saturated Fat 3.8g		19%
Trans Fat 0g		
Cholesterol 0mg		0%
Sodium 103mg		4%
Total Carbohydrates 6g		2%
Dietary Fiber 1g		2%
Sugars 4g		
Protein 1g		1%
Vitamin A 25% • Vitamin C 34%		
Calcium 3% • Iron		7%
* Percent Daily Values are based on 2000 calorie diet. Your Daily Values may be higher or lower depending on your calorie needs.		

COOKING INSTRUCTIONS:

1. In a salad bowl, mix the tempeh, chickpeas, capers, and onion.

2. In a small bowl, whisk the olive oil, vinegar, salt, and black pepper. Drizzle the mixture on the salad and toss well.

3. Serve immediately.

Zucchini Fennel Salad

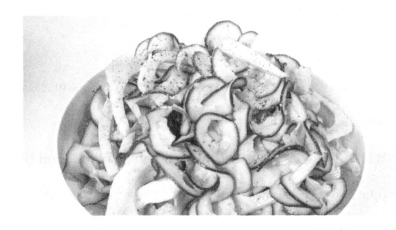

Total Time: 17 minutes | Servings: 4

INGREDIENTS:

2 lb. zucchinis cut into ½-inch cubes

2 tbsp vegan butter

Salt and black pepper to taste

2 oz. chopped scallions

3 oz. fennel, greenside sliced finely

1 cup vegan mayonnaise

2 tbsp fresh chives, finely chopped

A pinch mustard powder

Chopped dill to garnish

Nutrition Facts

Amount per
1 serving (12.1 oz)   342 g

Calories 333	From Fat 245
	% Daily Value*
Total Fat 27.4g	42%
Saturated Fat 6.1g	31%
Trans Fat 0.3g	
Cholesterol 27mg	9%
Sodium 536mg	22%
Total Carbohydrates 12g	4%
Dietary Fiber 4g	16%
Sugars 2g	
Protein 14g	28%

Vitamin A 34% • Vitamin C 180%
Calcium 10% • Iron 13%
* Percent Daily Values are based on 2000
calorie diet. Your Daily Values may be
higher or lower depending on your
calorie needs.

COOKING INSTRUCTIONS:

1. Heat the vegan butters in a medium skillet over medium heat and sauté the zucchinis until slightly softened but not browned, 7 minutes.

2. Turn off the heat, pour the zucchinis into a salad bowl and allow cooling.

3. Mix in the scallions, fennel, vegan mayonnaise, chives, and mustard powder.

4. Garnish with dill and serve.

Vegan Greek Salad

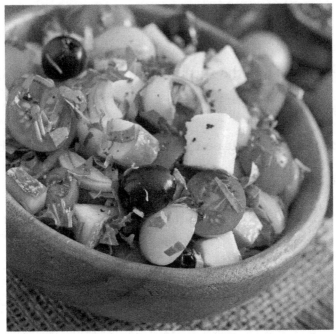

Total Time: 10 minutes | Servings: 2

INGREDIENTS:

For the salad:

½ yellow bell pepper, seeded and cut into bite-size pieces

½ red onion, peeled and sliced thinly

½ cup tofu cheese, cut into bite-size squares

10 Kalamata olives pitted

3 large tomatoes cut into bite-size pieces

Nutrition Facts		
Amount per 1 serving (8.2 oz)		233 g
Calories 254	From Fat	188
		% Daily Value*
Total Fat 21.4g		33%
Saturated Fat 6.1g		31%
Trans Fat 0g		
Cholesterol 17mg		6%
Sodium 610mg		25%
Total Carbohydrates 11g		4%
Dietary Fiber 3g		10%
Sugars 7g		
Protein 7g		14%
Vitamin A 32% • Vitamin C 101%		
Calcium 20% • Iron		6%
* Percent Daily Values are based on 2000 calorie diet. Your Daily Values may be higher or lower depending on your calorie needs.		

½ cucumber, cut into bite-size pieces

For the dressing:

4 tbsp olive oil

½ tbsp red wine vinegar

2 tsp dried oregano

Salt and black pepper to taste

COOKING INSTRUCTIONS:

1. In a salad bowl, combine all the salad's ingredients until well combined
2. In a small bowl, mix the dressing's ingredients and toss into the salad.
3. Dish the salad and enjoy!

Beet Tofu Salad

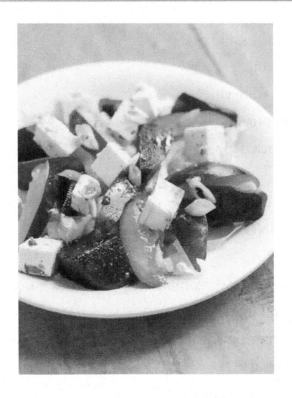

Total Time: 10 minutes | Servings: 4

INGREDIENTS:

2 tbsp vegan butter
2 oz. tofu, chopped into little bits
2 cups chopped steamed beets
½ red onion, sliced
1 cup vegan mayonnaise
1 small romaine lettuce, torn into small pieces
1 tbsp chopped fresh chives

Nutrition Facts

Amount per
1 serving (6.9 oz)   197 g

Calories 357	From Fat	247
		% Daily Value*
Total Fat 27.8g		43%
Saturated Fat 5.8g		29%
Trans Fat 0.3g		
Cholesterol 15mg		5%
Sodium 812mg		34%
Total Carbohydrates 22g		7%
Dietary Fiber 4g		17%
Sugars 16g		
Protein 7g		14%
Vitamin A 6% • Vitamin C		5%
Calcium 10% • Iron		7%

* Percent Daily Values are based on 2000 calorie diet. Your Daily Values may be higher or lower depending on your calorie needs.

COOKING INSTRUCTIONS:

1. Melt the vegan butter in a medium skillet over medium heat and fry the tofu until golden brown.

2. Transfer the tofu to a salad bowl and add the remaining ingredients.

3. Mix well and dish the salad.

4. Enjoy immediately!

Roasted Green Beans and Mushroom Salad

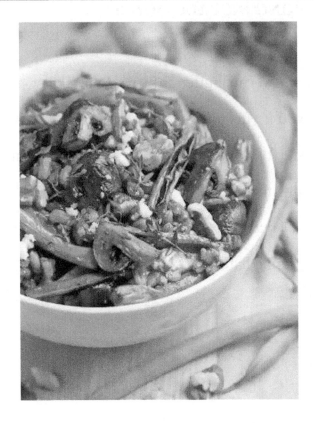

Total Time: 25 minutes | Servings: 4

INGREDIENTS:

½ cup green beans

1 lb. cremini mushrooms, sliced

3 tbsp melted vegan butter

Salt and black pepper to taste

1 lemon, juiced

4 tbsp toasted pecans

Nutrition Facts		
Amount per		
1 serving (6.1 oz)		173 g
Calories 473	From Fat	130
		% Daily Value*
Total Fat 15.1g		23%
Saturated Fat 6.3g		31%
Trans Fat 0.3g		
Cholesterol 23mg		8%
Sodium 112mg		5%
Total Carbohydrates 89g		30%
Dietary Fiber 14g		57%
Sugars 4g		
Protein 12g		24%
Vitamin A 9% • Vitamin C 61%		
Calcium 3% • Iron 14%		
* Percent Daily Values are based on 2000 calorie diet. Your Daily Values may be higher or lower depending on your calorie needs.		

COOKING INSTRUCTIONS:

1. Preheat the oven to 450 F.

2. Spread the green beans and mushrooms on a baking sheet, drizzle the vegan butter all over, and season with salt and black pepper. Rub the seasoning well onto the vegetables and roast in the oven for 20 minutes or until the vegetables soften.

3. Transfer the vegetables to a salad bowl, drizzle with the lemon juice, and toss the salad with the pecans.

4. Serve immediately.

Brussel Sprouts, Nuts & Seed Salad

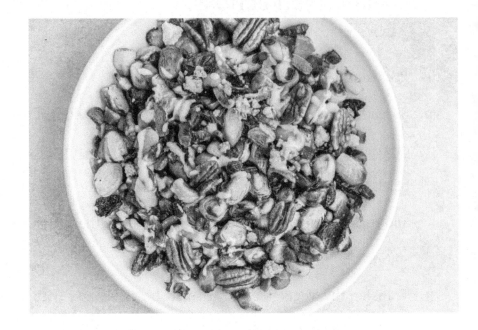

Total Time: 17 minutes | Servings: 4

INGREDIENTS:

1 lb Brussels sprouts, trimmed
½ cup olive oil
1 lemon, zested and juiced
Salt and black pepper to taste
1 tbsp vegan butter
1 tsp chili paste
2 oz. pecans
1 oz. pumpkin seeds
1 oz. sunflower seeds
½ tsp cumin powder
1 pinch salt

Nutrition Facts

Amount per
1 serving (6.9 oz)   197 g

Calories 494	From Fat 396

	% Daily Value*
Total Fat 45.7g	70%
Saturated Fat 7.1g	36%
Trans Fat 0.1g	
Cholesterol 8mg	3%
Sodium 74mg	3%
Total Carbohydrates 20g	7%
Dietary Fiber 8g	32%
Sugars 4g	
Protein 8g	17%

Vitamin A 26%	•	Vitamin C 214%
Calcium 8%	•	Iron 18%

* Percent Daily Values are based on 2000
calorie diet. Your Daily Values may be
higher or lower depending on your
calorie needs.

COOKING INSTRUCTIONS:

1. Place the Brussels sprouts in a food processor and shred coarsely. Transfer to a salad bowl.

2. In a small bowl, mix the olive oil, lemon zest, lemon juice, salt, black pepper, and drizzle the dressing over the Brussels sprouts. Toss and allow sitting for 10 minutes to marinate the vegetables.

3. Meanwhile, melt the vegan butter in a frying pan over low heat. Mix in the remaining ingredients until well coated with the butter and fragrant, 2 to 3 minutes.

4. Pour the nuts and seeds mix onto the Brussel sprouts and toss well.

5. Serve the salad.

Warm Collard Salad

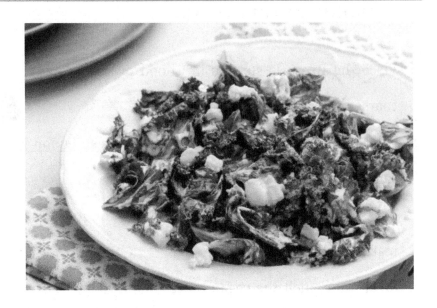

Total Time: 10 minutes | Servings: 2

INGREDIENTS:

¾ cup coconut whipping cream

2 tbsp coconut oil

1 tbsp. spirinula

1 garlic clove, minced

2 tbsp vegan mayonnaise

A pinch of mustard powder

Salt and black pepper to taste.

2 oz. vegan butter

1 cup collards, rinsed

4 oz. tofu cheese

Nutrition Facts		
Amount per		
1 serving (3.1 oz)		89 g
Calories 299	From Fat	252
	% Daily Value*	
Total Fat 29g		45%
Saturated Fat 15.8g		79%
Trans Fat 0.5g		
Cholesterol 39mg		13%
Sodium 157mg		7%
Total Carbohydrates 6g		2%
Dietary Fiber 2g		7%
Sugars 2g		
Protein 6g		13%
Vitamin A 21% • Vitamin C		51%
Calcium 15% • Iron		9%
* Percent Daily Values are based on 2000 calorie diet. Your Daily Values may be higher or lower depending on your calorie needs.		

COOKING INSTRUCTIONS:

1. In a small bowl, whisk the coconut whipping cream, coconut oil, spirinula, garlic, vegan mayonnaise, mustard powder, salt, and black pepper. Set aside.

2. Melt the vegan butter in a large skillet over medium heat and sauté the collards until wilted and slightly brown. Season with salt and black pepper to taste.

3. Transfer the collards to a salad bowl and pour the coconut cream dressing all over. Toss well and scatter the tofu cheese on top.

4. Serve the salad warm.

Fried Broccoli Salad with Seitan and Tangerine

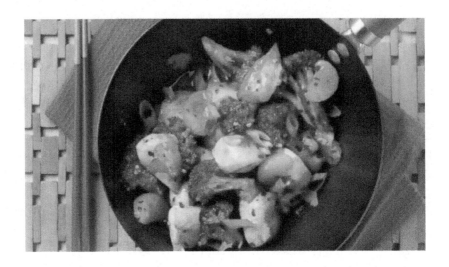

Total Time: 10 minutes | Servings: 11

INGREDIENTS:

3 oz. vegan butter

¾ lb. seitan slices cut into 1-inch cubes

1 lb broccoli florets

Salt and ground black pepper to taste

2 oz. almonds

½ cup tangerine segments, quartered

Nutrition Facts

Amount per
1 serving (3.1 oz)   89 g

Calories 299	From Fat 252

% Daily Value*

Total Fat 29g	45%
Saturated Fat 15.8g	79%
Trans Fat 0.5g	
Cholesterol 39mg	13%
Sodium 157mg	7%
Total Carbohydrates 6g	2%
Dietary Fiber 2g	7%
Sugars 2g	
Protein 6g	13%

Vitamin A 21%	• Vitamin C 51%
Calcium 15%	• Iron 9%

* Percent Daily Values are based on 2000
calorie diet. Your Daily Values may be
higher or lower depending on your
calorie needs.

COOKING INSTRUCTIONS:

1. In a deep skillet, melt the vegan butter over medium heat and fry the seitan until brown on all sides.

2. Mix in the broccoli and cook until softened, 5 minutes. Season with salt, black pepper, and turn the heat off.

3. Stir in the almonds, tangerine, and dish the salad.

4. Serve warm.

Soups

Medley of Mushroom Soup

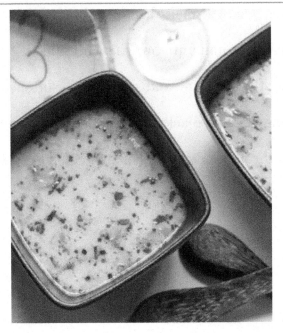

Total Time: 25 minutes | Servings: 4

INGREDIENTS:

4 oz. unsalted vegan butter

1 small onion, finely chopped

1 garlic clove, minced

2 cups sliced mixed mushrooms

½ lb celery root, chopped

½ tsp dried rosemary

3 cups of water

1 vegan stock cube, crushed

1 tbsp plain vinegar

1 cup coconut cream

6 leaves basil, chopped

Nutrition Facts		
Amount per		
1 serving (13.4 oz)		380 g
Calories 743	From Fat	540
		% Daily Value*
Total Fat 62.7g		97%
Saturated Fat 15.8g		79%
Trans Fat 0.6g		
Cholesterol 37mg		12%
Sodium 653mg		27%
Total Carbohydrates 28g		9%
Dietary Fiber 7g		28%
Sugars 7g		
Protein 27g		54%
Vitamin A 18% • Vitamin C		71%
Calcium 18% • Iron		37%
* Percent Daily Values are based on 2,000 calorie diet. Your Daily Values may be higher or lower depending on your calorie needs.		

COOKING INSTRUCTIONS:

1. Melt the vegan butter in a medium pot and sauté the onion, garlic, mushrooms, celery, and rosemary until the vegetables soften, 5 minutes.

2. Stir in the water, stock cube, and vinegar. Cover the pot, allow boiling, and then, simmer for 10 minutes.

3. Mix in the coconut cream and puree the ingredients using an immersion blender until smooth. Simmer for 2 minutes.

4. Dish the soup and serve warm.

Spinach and Kale Soup

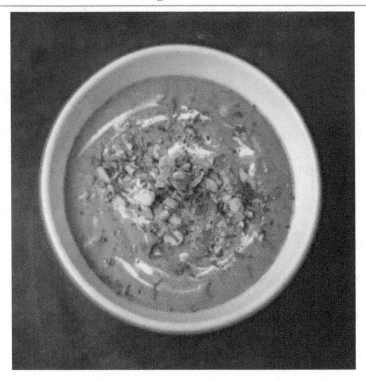

Total Time: 10 minutes | Servings: 2

INGREDIENTS:

For the soup:

3 oz. vegan butter

1 cup fresh spinach, chopped coarsely

1 cup fresh kale, chopped coarsely

1 large avocado

3 tbsp chopped fresh mint leaves

3 ½ cups coconut cream

1 cup vegetable broth

Salt and black pepper to taste

1 lime, juiced

Nutrition Facts		
Amount per		
1 serving (13.4 oz)		380 g
Calories 743	From Fat	540
		% Daily Value*
Total Fat 62.7g		97%
Saturated Fat 15.8g		79%
Trans Fat 0.6g		
Cholesterol 37mg		12%
Sodium 653mg		27%
Total Carbohydrates 28g		9%
Dietary Fiber 7g		28%
Sugars 7g		
Protein 27g		54%
Vitamin A 18% • Vitamin C 71%		
Calcium 18% • Iron 37%		
* Percent Daily Values are based on 2000 calorie diet. Your Daily Values may be higher or lower depending on your calorie needs.		

COOKING INSTRUCTIONS:

1. Melt the vegan butter in a medium pot over medium heat and sauté the kale and spinach until wilted, 3 minutes. Turn the heat off.

2. Stir in the remaining ingredients and using an immersion blender, puree the soup until smooth.

3. Dish the soup and serve warm.

Coconut and Grilled Vegetable Soup

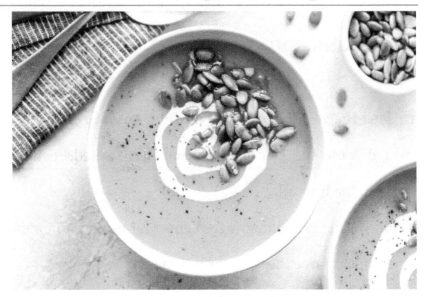

Total Time: 55 minutes | Servings: 4

INGREDIENTS:

2 small red onions cut into wedges
2 garlic cloves
10 oz. butternut squash, peeled and chopped
10 oz. pumpkins, peeled and chopped
4 tbsp melted vegan butter
Salt and black pepper to taste
1 cup of water
1 cup unsweetened coconut milk
1 lime juiced
¾ cup vegan mayonnaise
Toasted pumpkin seeds for garnishing

Nutrition Facts

Amount per
1 serving (13.6 oz)   387 g

Calories 1672	From Fat 1571
	% Daily Value*
Total Fat 181.9g	280%
Saturated Fat 144.7g	724%
Trans Fat 0.7g	
Cholesterol 54mg	18%
Sodium 696mg	29%
Total Carbohydrates 12g	4%
Dietary Fiber 4g	15%
Sugars 7g	
Protein 15g	29%

Vitamin A 60%	Vitamin C 36%
Calcium 36%	Iron 12%

* Percent Daily Values are based on 2000
calorie diet. Your Daily Values may be
higher or lower depending on your
calorie needs.

COOKING INSTRUCTIONS:

1. Preheat the oven to 400 F.

2. On a baking sheet, spread the onions, garlic, butternut squash, and pumpkins and drizzle half of the butter on top. Season with salt, black pepper, and rub the seasoning well onto the vegetables. Roast in the oven for 45 minutes or until the vegetables are golden brown and softened.

3. Transfer the vegetables to a pot; add the remaining ingredients except for the pumpkin seeds and using an immersion blender puree the ingredients until smooth.

4. Dish the soup, garnish with the pumpkin seeds and serve warm.

Celery Dill Soup

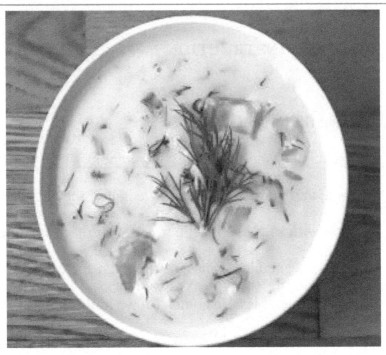

Total Time: 30 minutes | Servings: 4

INGREDIENTS:

2 tbsp coconut oil

½ lb celery root, trimmed

1 garlic clove

1 medium white onion

¼ cup fresh dill, roughly chopped

1 tsp cumin powder

¼ tsp nutmeg powder

1 small head cauliflower, cut into florets

3½ cups seasoned vegetable stock

5 oz. vegan butter

Juice from 1 lemon

Nutrition Facts		
Amount per		
1 serving (14.9 oz)		424 g
Calories 2055	**From Fat** 2004	
		% Daily Value*
Total Fat 232.1g		357%
Saturated Fat 184.4g		922%
Trans Fat 1.2g		
Cholesterol 76mg		25%
Sodium 297mg		12%
Total Carbohydrates 11g		4%
Dietary Fiber 3g		13%
Sugars 4g		
Protein 3g		7%
Vitamin A 26% • **Vitamin C** 115%		
Calcium 6% • **Iron** 8%		
* Percent Daily Values are based on 2000 calorie diet. Your Daily Values may be higher or lower depending on your calorie needs.		

¼ cup coconut cream

Salt and black pepper to taste

COOKING INSTRUCTIONS:

1. Melt the coconut oil in a large pot and sauté the celery root, garlic, and onion until softened and fragrant, 5 minutes.

2. Stir in the dill, cumin, and nutmeg, and stir-fry for 1 minute. Mix in the cauliflower and vegetable stock. Allow the soup to boil for 15 minutes and turn the heat off.

3. Add the vegan butter and lemon juice, and puree the soup using an immersion blender.

4. Stir in the coconut cream, salt, black pepper, and dish the soup.

5. Serve warm.

Broccoli Fennel Soup

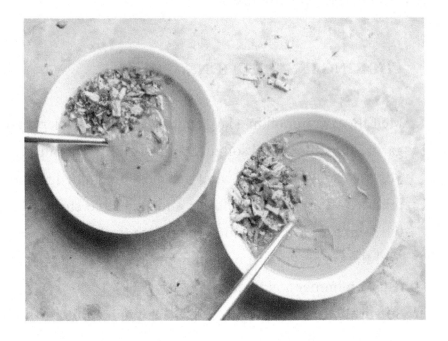

Total Time: 30 minutes | Servings: 4

INGREDIENTS:

1 fennel bulb, white and green parts coarsely chopped
10 oz. broccoli, cut into florets
3 cups vegetable stock
Salt and freshly ground black pepper
1 garlic clove
1 cup dairy-free cream cheese
3 oz. vegan butter
½ cup chopped fresh oregano

Nutrition Facts		
Amount per		
1 serving (12.7 oz)		359 g
Calories 1690	From Fat 1629	
		% Daily Value*
Total Fat 188.5g		290%
Saturated Fat 148.8g		744%
Trans Fat 1g		
Cholesterol 65mg		22%
Sodium 208mg		9%
Total Carbohydrates 15g		5%
Dietary Fiber 3g		14%
Sugars 5g		
Protein 2g		5%
Vitamin A 159% • Vitamin C 108%		
Calcium 6% • Iron		8%
*Percent Daily Values are based on 2000 calorie diet. Your Daily Values may be higher or lower depending on your calorie needs.		

COOKING INSTRUCTIONS:

1. In a medium pot, combine the fennel, broccoli, vegetable stock, salt, and black pepper. Bring to a boil until the vegetables soften, 10 to 15 minutes.

2. Stir in the remaining ingredients and simmer the soup for 3 to 5 minutes.

3. Adjust the taste with salt and black pepper, and dish the soup.

4. Serve warm.

Tofu Goulash Soup

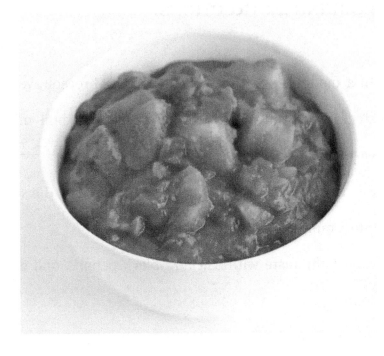

Total Time: 55 minutes | Servings: 4

INGREDIENTS:

4¼ oz. vegan butter

1 white onion, chopped

2 garlic cloves, minced

1 ½ cups butternut squash

1 red bell pepper, deseeded and chopped

1 tbsp paprika powder

¼ tsp red chili flakes

1 tbsp dried basil

½ tbsp crushed cardamom seeds

Salt and black pepper to taste

1 ½ cups crushed tomatoes

Nutrition Facts		
Amount per		
1 serving (12.3 oz)		349 g
Calories 358	From Fat	316
		% Daily Value*
Total Fat 36.6g		56%
Saturated Fat 28.2g		141%
Trans Fat 0g		
Cholesterol 30mg		10%
Sodium 63mg		3%
Total Carbohydrates 8g		3%
Dietary Fiber 3g		10%
Sugars 2g		
Protein 4g		8%
Vitamin A 16% • Vitamin C		9%
Calcium 7% • Iron		11%
* Percent Daily Values are based on 2000 calorie diet. Your Daily Values may be higher or lower depending on your calorie needs.		

3 cups vegetable broth
1½ tsp red wine vinegar
Chopped parsley to serve

COOKING INSTRUCTIONS:

1. Place the tofu between two paper towels and allow draining of water for 30 minutes. After, crumble the tofu and set aside.
2. Melt the vegan butter in a large pot over medium heat and sauté the onion and garlic until the veggies are fragrant and soft, 3 minutes.
3. Stir in the tofu and cook until golden brown, 3 minutes.
4. Add the butternut squash, bell pepper, paprika, red chili flakes, basil, cardamom seeds, salt, and black pepper. Cook for 2 minutes to release some flavor and mix in the tomatoes and 2 cups of vegetable broth.
5. Close the lid, bring the soup to a boil, and then simmer for 10 minutes.
6. Stir in the remaining vegetable broth, the red wine vinegar, and adjust the taste with salt and black pepper.
7. Dish the soup, garnish with the parsley and serve warm.

Tofu and Mushroom Soup

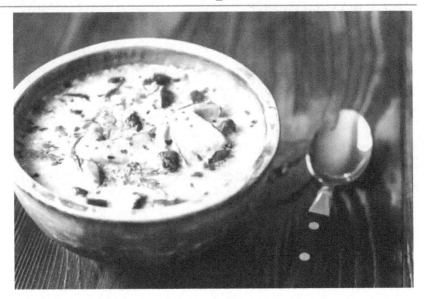

Total Time: 25 minutes | Servings: 4

INGREDIENTS:

2 tbsp olive oil

1 garlic clove, minced

1 large yellow onion, finely chopped

1 tsp freshly grated ginger

1 cup vegetable stock

2 small potatoes, peeled and chopped

¼ tsp salt

¼ tsp black pepper

2 (14 oz) silken tofu, drained and rinsed

2/3 cup baby Bella mushrooms, sliced

1 tbsp chopped fresh oregano

2 tbsp chopped fresh parsley to garnish

Nutrition Facts		
Amount per		
1 serving (17.1 oz)		484 g
Calories 525	**From Fat**	235
		% Daily Value*
Total Fat 26.6g		41%
Saturated Fat 11.1g		56%
Trans Fat 0g		
Cholesterol 45mg		15%
Sodium 771mg		32%
Total Carbohydrates 41g		14%
Dietary Fiber 5g		21%
Sugars 5g		
Protein 33g		65%
Vitamin A 11% • **Vitamin C** 71%		
Calcium 65% • **Iron** 21%		
* Percent Daily Values are based on 2000 calorie diet. Your Daily Values may be higher or lower depending on your calorie needs.		

COOKING INSTRUCTIONS:

1. Heat the olive oil in a medium pot over medium heat and sauté the garlic, onion, and ginger until soft and fragrant.

2. Pour in the vegetable stock, potatoes, salt, and black pepper. Cook until the potatoes soften, 12 minutes.

3. Stir in the tofu and using an immersion blender, puree the ingredients until smooth.

4. Mix in the mushrooms and simmer with the pot covered until the mushrooms warm up while occasionally stirring to ensure that the tofu doesn't curdle, 7 minutes.

5. Stir oregano, and dish the soup.

6. Garnish with the parsley and serve warm.

Avocado Green Soup

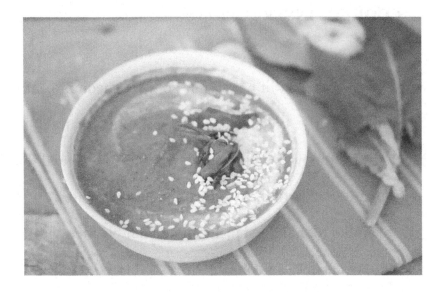

Total Time: 10 minutes | Servings: 4

INGREDIENTS:

2 tbsp olive oil

1 ½ cup fresh kale, chopped coarsely

1 ½ cup fresh spinach, chopped coarsely

3 large avocados, halved, pitted and pulp extracted

2 cups of soy milk

2 cups no-sodium vegetable broth

3 tbsp chopped fresh mint leaves

¼ tsp salt

¼ tsp black pepper

2 limes, juiced

Nutrition Facts

Amount per
1 serving (15.2 oz)   431 g

Calories 635	From Fat 421

% Daily Value*

Total Fat 48.5g	75%
Saturated Fat 15.8g	79%
Trans Fat 0g	
Cholesterol 69mg	23%
Sodium 614mg	26%
Total Carbohydrates 29g	10%
Dietary Fiber 11g	43%
Sugars 12g	
Protein 27g	54%

Vitamin A 53% • Vitamin C	54%
Calcium 29% • Iron	9%

* Percent Daily Values are based on 2000
calorie diet. Your Daily Values may be
higher or lower depending on your
calorie needs.

COOKING INSTRUCTIONS:

1. Heat the olive oil in a medium saucepan over medium heat and mix in the kale and spinach. Cook until wilted, 3 minutes and turn off the heat.

2. Add the remaining ingredients and using an immersion blender, puree the soup until smooth.

3. Dish the soup and serve immediately.

Cucumber Dill Gazpacho

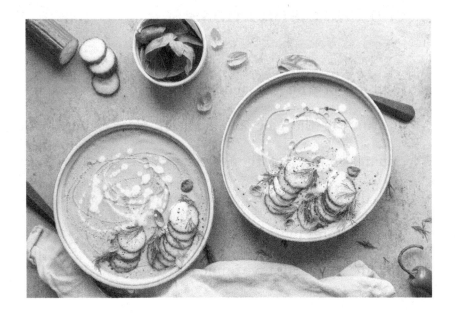

Time: 2 hours 10 minutes | Servings: 4

INGREDIENTS:

4 large cucumbers, peeled, deseeded, and chopped

1/8 tsp salt

1 tsp chopped fresh dill + more for garnishing

2 tbsp freshly squeezed lemon juice

1 ½ cups green grape, seeds removed

3 tbsp extra virgin olive oil

1 garlic clove, minced

Nutrition Facts		
Amount per		
1 serving (12.6 oz)		357 g
Calories 118	From Fat	46
		% Daily Value*
Total Fat 5.1g		8%
Saturated Fat 0.7g		3%
Trans Fat 0g		
Cholesterol 4mg		1%
Sodium 175mg		7%
Total Carbohydrates 17g		6%
Dietary Fiber 3g		10%
Sugars 13g		
Protein 2g		5%
Vitamin A 5% • **Vitamin C** 24%		
Calcium 6% • **Iron** 5%		
* Percent Daily Values are based on 2000 calorie diet. Your Daily Values may be higher or lower depending on your calorie needs.		

COOKING INSTRUCTIONS:

1. Add all the ingredients to a food processor and blend until smooth.

2. Pour the soup into serving bowls and chill for 1 to 2 hours.

3. Garnish with dill and serve chilled.

Potato Leek Soup

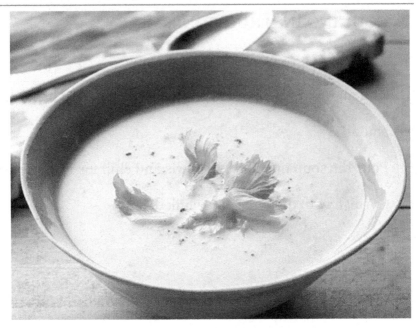

Time: 5 minutes | Servings: 4

INGREDIENTS:

1 cup fresh cilantro leaves

6 garlic cloves, peeled

3 tbsp vegetable oil

3 leeks, white and green parts chopped

2 lb russet potatoes, peeled and chopped

1 tsp cumin powder

¼ tsp salt

¼ tsp black pepper

2 bay leaves

6 cups no-sodium vegetable broth

Nutrition Facts

Amount per	
1 serving (12.6 oz)	357 g

Calories 118	From Fat 46
	% Daily Value*

	% Daily Value*
Total Fat 5.1g	8%
Saturated Fat 0.7g	3%
Trans Fat 0g	
Cholesterol 4mg	1%
Sodium 175mg	7%
Total Carbohydrates 17g	6%
Dietary Fiber 3g	10%
Sugars 13g	
Protein 2g	5%

Vitamin A 5% • Vitamin C 24%
Calcium 6% • Iron 5%

* Percent Daily Values are based on 2000 calorie diet. Your Daily Values may be higher or lower depending on your calorie needs.

COOKING INSTRUCTIONS:

1. In a spice blender, process the cilantro and garlic until smooth paste forms.

2. Heat the vegetable oil in a large pot and sauté the garlic mixture and leeks until the leeks are tender, 5 minutes.

3. Mix in the remaining ingredients and allow boiling until the potatoes soften, 15 minutes.

4. Turn the heat off, open the lid, remove and discard the bay leaves.

5. Using an immersion blender, puree the soup until smooth.

6. Dish the food and serve warm.

Noodles Alfredo with Herby Tofu

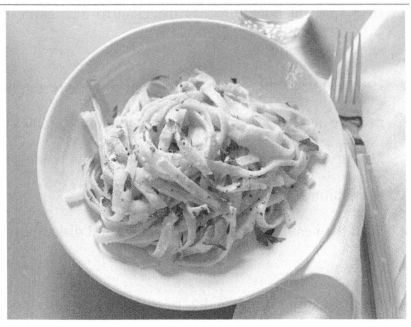

Time: 10 minutes | Servings: 4

INGREDIENTS:

2 tbsp vegetable oil

2 (14 oz.) blocks extra-firm tofu, pressed and cubed

12 ounces eggless noodles

1 tbsp dried mixed herbs

2 cups cashews, soaked overnight and drained

¾ cups unsweetened almond milk

½ cup nutritional yeast

Nutrition Facts		
Amount per		
1 serving (12.9 oz)		367 g
Calories 391	From Fat	181
		% Daily Value*
Total Fat 21.2g		33%
Saturated Fat 2.3g		12%
Trans Fat 0g		
Cholesterol 0mg		0%
Sodium 1135mg		47%
Total Carbohydrates 24g		8%
Dietary Fiber 5g		19%
Sugars 10g		
Protein 33g		66%
Vitamin A 6% • Vitamin C 66%		
Calcium 53% • Iron 37%		
* Percent Daily Values are based on 2000 calorie diet. Your Daily Values may be higher or lower depending on your calorie needs.		

4 garlic cloves, roasted (roasting is optional but highly recommended)
½ cup onion, coarsely chopped
1 lemon, juiced
½ cup sun-dried tomatoes
Salt and black pepper to taste
2 tbsp chopped fresh basil leaves to garnish

COOKING INSTRUCTIONS:

1. Heat the vegetable oil in a large skillet over medium heat.

2. Season the tofu with the mixed herbs, salt, black pepper, and fry in the oil until golden brown. Transfer to a paper-towel-lined plate and set aside. Turn the heat off.

3. In a blender, combine the almond milk, nutritional yeast, garlic, onion, and lemon juice. Set aside.

4. Reheat the vegetable oil in the skillet over medium heat and sauté the noodles for 2 minutes. Stir in the sundried tomatoes and the cashew (Alfredo) sauce. Reduce the heat to low and cook for 2 more minutes.

5. If the sauce is too thick, thin with some more almond milk to your desired thickness.

6. Dish the food, garnish with the basil and serve warm.

Lemon Couscous with Tempeh Kabobs

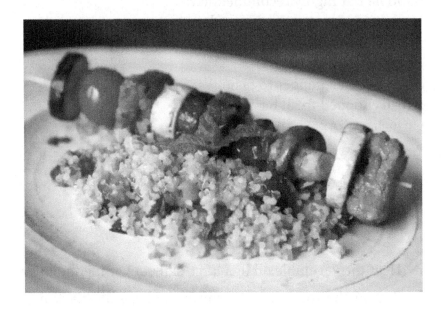

Time: 2 hours 15 minutes | Servings: 4

INGREDIENTS:

For the tempeh kabobs:
1 ½ cups of water
10 oz. tempeh, cut into 1-inch chunks
1 red onion, cut into 1-inch chunks
1 small yellow squash, cut into 1-inch chunks
1 small green squash, cut into 1-inch chunks
2 tbsp. olive oil
1 cup sugar-free barbecue sauce
8 wooden skewers, soaked

For the lemon couscous:
1 ½ cups whole wheat couscous
2 cups of water

Nutrition Facts		
Amount per		
1 serving (20.2 oz)		573 g
Calories 392	From Fat	199
		% Daily Value*
Total Fat 23.4g		36%
Saturated Fat 4g		20%
Trans Fat 0g		
Cholesterol 8mg		3%
Sodium 51mg		2%
Total Carbohydrates 32g		11%
Dietary Fiber 6g		25%
Sugars 4g		
Protein 21g		42%
Vitamin A 12% • Vitamin C		78%
Calcium 14% • Iron		19%
* Percent Daily Values are based on 2000 calorie diet. Your Daily Values may be higher or lower depending on your calorie needs.		

Salt to taste
¼ cup chopped parsley
¼ chopped mint leaves
¼ cup chopped cilantro
1 lemon, juiced
1 medium avocado, pitted, sliced and
peeled

COOKING INSTRUCTIONS:

For the tempeh kabobs:
1. Boil the water in a medium pot over medium heat.
2. Once boiled, turn the heat off, and put the tempeh in it. Cover the lid and let the tempeh steam for 5 minutes (this is to remove its bitterness). Drain the tempeh after.
3. After, pour the barbecue sauce into a medium bowl, add the tempeh, and coat well with the sauce. Cover the bowl with plastic wrap and marinate for 2 hours.
4. After 2 hours, preheat a grill to 350 F.
5. On the skewers, alternately thread single chunks of the tempeh, onion, yellow squash, and green squash until the ingredients are exhausted.
6. Lightly grease the grill grates with olive oil, place the skewers on top and brush with some barbecue sauce. Cook for 3 minutes on each side while brushing with more barbecue sauce as you turn the kabobs.
7. Transfer to a plate for serving.

For the lemon couscous:
8. Meanwhile, as the kabobs cooked, pour the couscous, water, and salt into a medium bowl and steam in the microwave for 3 to 4 minutes. Remove the bowl from the microwave and allow slight cooling.
9. Stir in the parsley, mint leaves, cilantro, and lemon juice.
10. Garnish the couscous with the avocado slices and serve with the tempeh kabobs.

Portobello Burger with Veggie Fries

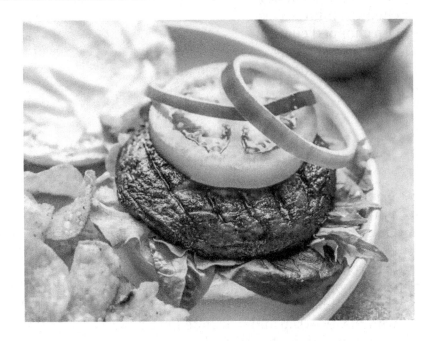

Time: 45 minutes | Servings: 4

INGREDIENTS:
For the veggie fries:
3 carrots, peeled and julienned
2 sweet potatoes, peeled and julienned
1 rutabaga, peeled and julienned
2 tsp olive oil
¼ tsp paprika
Salt and black pepper to taste

For the Portobello burgers:
1 clove garlic, minced
½ tsp salt
2 tbsp. olive oil
4 whole-wheat buns

Nutrition Facts		
Amount per		
1 serving (14.2 oz)		402 g
Calories 757	From Fat	606
		% Daily Value*
Total Fat 67.6g		104%
Saturated Fat 10.4g		52%
Trans Fat 0g		
Cholesterol 57mg		19%
Sodium 1581mg		66%
Total Carbohydrates 32g		11%
Dietary Fiber 6g		24%
Sugars 17g		
Protein 8g		15%
Vitamin A 144% • Vitamin C 155%		
Calcium 17% • Iron		12%
* Percent Daily Values are based on 2000 calorie diet. Your Daily Values may be higher or lower depending on your calorie needs.		

4 Portobello mushroom caps
½ cup sliced roasted red peppers
2 tbsp. pitted Kalamata olives,
chopped
2 medium tomatoes, chopped
½ tsp dried oregano
¼ cup crumbled feta cheese
(optional)
1 tbsp. red wine vinegar
2 cups baby salad greens
½ cup hummus for serving

COOKING INSTRUCTIONS:

For the veggie fries:

1. Preheat the oven to 400 F.
2. Spread the carrots, sweet potatoes, and rutabaga on a baking sheet and season with the olive oil, paprika, salt, and black pepper. Use your hands to rub the seasoning well onto the vegetables. Bake in the oven for 20 minutes or until the vegetables soften (stir halfway).
3. When ready, transfer to a plate and use it for serving.
For the Portobello burgers:
4. Meanwhile, as the vegetable roast, heat a grill pan over medium heat.
5. Use a spoon to crush the garlic with salt in a bowl. Stir in 1 tablespoon of the olive oil.
6. Brush the mushrooms on both sides with the garlic mixture and grill in the pan on both sides until tender, 8 minutes. Transfer to a plate and set aside.
7. Toast the buns in the pan until crispy, 2 minutes. Set aside in a plate.
8. In a bowl, combine the remaining ingredients except for the hummus and divide on the bottom parts of the buns.
9. Top with the hummus, cover the burger with the top parts of the buns and serve with the veggie fries.

Thai Seitan Vegetable Curry

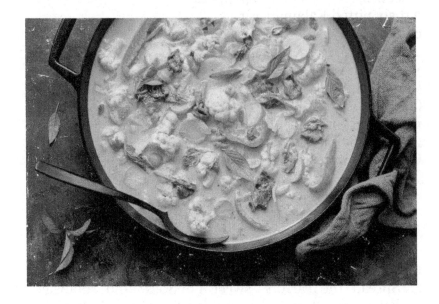

Time: 20 minutes | Servings: 4

INGREDIENTS:

1 tbsp vegetable oil

4 cups diced seitan

1 cup sliced mixed bell peppers

½ cup onions diced

1 small head broccoli, cut into florets

2 tbsp Thai red curry paste

1 tsp garlic puree

1 cup unsweetened coconut milk

2 tbsp vegetable broth

2 cups spinach

Salt and black pepper to taste

Nutrition Facts		
Amount per		
1 serving (4.5 oz)		127 g
Calories 155	From Fat	111
		% Daily Value*
Total Fat 12.8g		20%
Saturated Fat 7.3g		36%
Trans Fat 0g		
Cholesterol 6mg		2%
Sodium 42mg		2%
Total Carbohydrates 9g		3%
Dietary Fiber 3g		10%
Sugars 5g		
Protein 3g		7%
Vitamin A 35% • Vitamin C 100%		
Calcium 11% • Iron		7%
* Percent Daily Values are based on 2000 calorie diet. Your Daily Values may be higher or lower depending on your calorie needs.		

COOKING INSTRUCTIONS:

1. Heat the vegetable oil in a large skillet over medium heat and fry the seitan until slightly dark brown. Mix in the bell peppers, onions, broccoli, and cook until softened, 4 minutes.

2. Mix the curry paste, garlic puree, and 1 tablespoon of coconut milk. Cook for 1 minute and stir in the remaining coconut milk and vegetable broth. Simmer for 10 minutes.

3. Stir in the spinach to wilt and season the curry with salt and black pepper.

4. Serve the curry with steamed white or brown rice.

Tofu Cabbage Stir-Fry

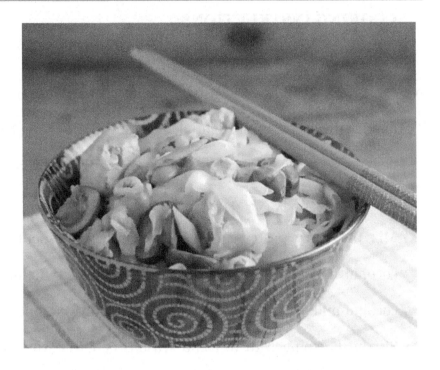

Time: 15 minutes | Servings: 4

INGREDIENTS:

5 oz. vegan butter

2 ½ cups baby bok choy, quartered lengthwise

8 oz sliced mushrooms

2 cups extra-firm tofu, pressed and cubed

Salt and black pepper to taste

1 tsp onion powder

1 tsp garlic powder

1 tbsp plain vinegar

2 garlic cloves, minced

Nutrition Facts		
Amount per		
1 serving (9 oz)		256 g
Calories 679	From Fat	548
		% Daily Value*
Total Fat 62.4g		96%
Saturated Fat 22.1g		110%
Trans Fat 1.3g		
Cholesterol 76mg		25%
Sodium 733mg		31%
Total Carbohydrates 11g		4%
Dietary Fiber 5g		18%
Sugars 2g		
Protein 25g		49%
Vitamin A 31% • Vitamin C		51%
Calcium 92% • Iron		23%
* Percent Daily Values are based on 2000 calorie diet. Your Daily Values may be higher or lower depending on your calorie needs.		

1 tsp chili flakes
1 tbsp fresh ginger, grated
3 scallions, sliced
1 tbsp sesame oil
1 cup vegan mayonnaise
Wasabi paste to taste
Cooked white or brown rice (1/2 cup per person)

COOKING INSTRUCTIONS:

1. Melt half of the vegan butter in a wok and sauté the bok choy until softened, 3 minutes.

2. Season with salt, black pepper, onion powder, garlic powder, and vinegar. Sauté for 2 minutes to combine the flavors and plate the bok choy.

3. Melt the remaining vegan butter in the wok and sauté the garlic, mushrooms, chili flakes, and ginger until fragrant.

4. Stir in the tofu and cook until browned on all sides. Add the scallions and bok choy, heat for 2 minutes and drizzle in the sesame oil.

5. In a small bowl, mix the vegan mayonnaise and wasabi, and mix into the tofu and vegetables. Cook for 2 minutes and dish the food.

6. Serve warm with steamed rice.

Curried Tofu with Buttery Cabbage

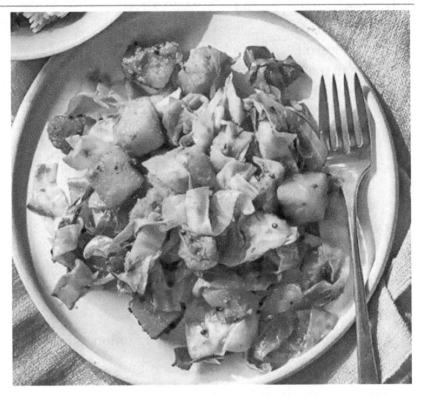

Time: 15 minutes | Servings: 4

INGREDIENTS:

2 cups extra-firm tofu, pressed and cubed

1 tbsp + 3 ½ tbsp coconut oil

½ cup unsweetened shredded coconut

1 tsp yellow curry powder

1 tsp salt

½ tsp onion powder

2 cups Napa cabbage

4 oz. vegan butter

Nutrition Facts		
Amount per		
1 serving (9.4 oz)		268 g
Calories 437	From Fat	326
		% Daily Value*
Total Fat 37.7g		58%
Saturated Fat 19.2g		96%
Trans Fat 0.9g		
Cholesterol 61mg		20%
Sodium 820mg		34%
Total Carbohydrates 10g		3%
Dietary Fiber 4g		15%
Sugars 2g		
Protein 21g		43%
Vitamin A 24% • **Vitamin C** 58%		
Calcium 90% • **Iron** 23%		
* Percent Daily Values are based on 2000 calorie diet. Your Daily Values may be higher or lower depending on your calorie needs.		

Salt and black pepper to taste

Lemon wedges for serving

COOKING INSTRUCTIONS:

1. In a medium bowl, add the tofu, 1 tablespoon of coconut oil, curry powder, salt, and onion powder. Mix well until the tofu is well-coated with the spices.

2. Heat the remaining coconut oil in a non-stick skillet and fry the tofu until golden brown on all sides, 8 minutes. Divide onto serving plates and set aside for serving.

3. In another skillet, melt half of the vegan butter, and sauté the cabbage until slightly caramelized, 2 minutes. Season with salt, black pepper, and plate to the side of the tofu.

4. Melt the remaining vegan butter in the skillet and drizzle all over the cabbage.

5. Serve warm.

Smoked Tempeh with Broccoli Fritters

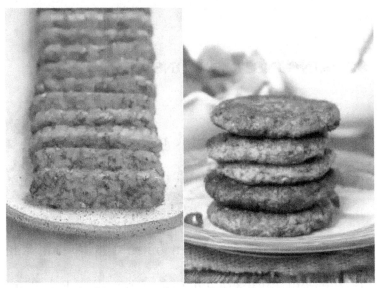

Time: 25 minutes | Servings: 4

INGREDIENTS:

For the flax egg:
4 tbsp flax seed powder + 12 tbsp water

For the grilled tempeh:
3 tbsp olive oil
1 tbsp soy sauce
3 tbsp fresh lime juice
1 tbsp grated ginger
Salt and cayenne pepper to taste
10 oz. tempeh slices

For the broccoli fritters:
2 cups of rice broccoli
8 oz. tofu cheese
3 tbsp plain flour
½ tsp onion powder

Nutrition Facts		
Amount per		
1 serving (11.3 oz)		321 g
Calories 968	From Fat	763
	% Daily Value*	
Total Fat 86.9g		134%
Saturated Fat 23.8g		119%
Trans Fat 1.1g		
Cholesterol 77mg		26%
Sodium 1588mg		66%
Total Carbohydrates 26g		9%
Dietary Fiber 4g		16%
Sugars 6g		
Protein 29g		58%
Vitamin A 29% • **Vitamin C** 62%		
Calcium 37% • **Iron** 33%		
* Percent Daily Values are based on 2000 calorie diet. Your Daily Values may be higher or lower depending on your calorie needs.		

1 tsp salt
¼ tsp freshly ground black pepper
4¼ oz. vegan butter

For serving:
½ cup mixed salad greens
1 cup vegan mayonnaise
½ lemon, juiced

COOKING INSTRUCTIONS:

For the smoked tempeh:
1. In a bowl, mix the flax seed powder with water and set aside to soak for 5 minutes.
2. In another bowl, combine the olive oil, soy sauce, lime juice, grated ginger, salt, and cayenne pepper. Brush the tempeh slices with the mixture.
3. Heat a grill pan over medium heat and grill the tempeh on both sides until nicely smoked and golden brown, 8 minutes. Transfer to a plate and set aside in a warmer for serving.
4. In a medium bowl, combine the broccoli rice, tofu cheese, flour, onion, salt, and black pepper. Mix in the flax egg until well combine and form 1-inch thick patties out of the mixture.
5. Melt the vegan butter in a medium skillet over medium heat and fry the patties on both sides until golden brown, 8 minutes. Remove the fritters onto a plate and set aside.
6. In a small bowl, mix the vegan mayonnaise with the lemon juice.
7. Divide the smoked tempeh and broccoli fritters onto serving plates, add the salad greens, and serve with the vegan mayonnaise sauce.

Cheesy Potato Casserole

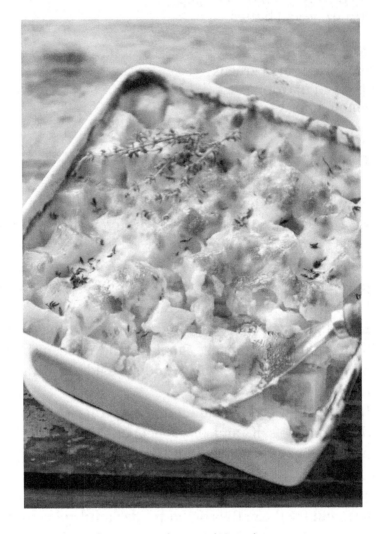

Time: 30 minutes | Servings: 4

INGREDIENTS:

2 oz. vegan butter

½ cup celery stalks, finely chopped

1 white onion, finely chopped

1 green bell pepper, seeded and finely chopped

Salt and black pepper to taste

2 cups peeled and chopped potatoes

1 cup vegan mayonnaise

4 oz. freshly shredded vegan Parmesan cheese

1 tsp red chili flakes

Nutrition Facts	
Amount per	
1 serving (8.5 oz)	241 g
Calories 480	**From Fat** 287
	% Daily Value*
Total Fat 32.2g	49%
Saturated Fat 10g	50%
Trans Fat 0.6g	
Cholesterol 36mg	12%
Sodium 903mg	38%
Total Carbohydrates 31g	10%
Dietary Fiber 3g	13%
Sugars 4g	
Protein 17g	35%
Vitamin A 15% • **Vitamin C** 120%	
Calcium 29% • **Iron** 14%	
* Percent Daily Values are based on 2000 calorie diet. Your Daily Values may be higher or lower depending on your calorie needs.	

COOKING INSTRUCTIONS:

1. Preheat the oven to 400 F and grease a baking dish with cooking spray.

2. Season the celery, onion, and bell pepper with salt and black pepper.

3. In a bowl, mix the potatoes, vegan mayonnaise, Parmesan cheese, and red chili flakes.

4. Pour the mixture into the baking dish, add the season vegetables, and mix well.

5. Bake in the oven until golden brown, about 20 minutes.

6. Remove the baked potato and serve warm with baby spinach.

Curry Mushroom Pie

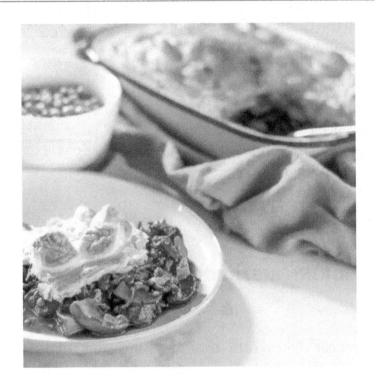

Time: 65 minutes | Servings: 4

INGREDIENTS:

For the piecrust:

1 tbsp flax seed powder + 3 tbsp water

¾ cup plain flour

4 tbsp. chia seeds

4 tbsp almond flour

1 tbsp nutritional yeast

1 tsp baking powder

1 pinch salt

3 tbsp olive oil

4 tbsp water

Nutrition Facts		
Amount per		
1 serving (7.6 oz)		215 g
Calories 587	From Fat	368
		% Daily Value*
Total Fat 41.9g		65%
Saturated Fat 13.3g		66%
Trans Fat 0.1g		
Cholesterol 5mg		2%
Sodium 890mg		37%
Total Carbohydrates 35g		12%
Dietary Fiber 3g		13%
Sugars 2g		
Protein 19g		39%
Vitamin A 6% • Vitamin C 25%		
Calcium 25% • Iron 21%		
* Percent Daily Values are based on 2000 calorie diet. Your Daily Values may be higher or lower depending on your calorie needs.		

For the filling:
1 cup chopped baby Bella mushrooms
1 cup vegan mayonnaise
3 tbsp + 9 tbsp water
½ red bell pepper, finely chopped
1 tsp curry powder
½ tsp paprika powder
½ tsp garlic powder
¼ tsp black pepper
½ cup coconut cream
1¼ cups shredded vegan Parmesan cheese

COOKING INSTRUCTIONS:

1. In two separate bowls, mix the different portions of flaxseed powder with the respective quantity of water. Allow soaking for 5 minutes.
   For the piecrust:
2. Preheat the oven to 350 F.
3. When the flax egg is ready, pour the smaller quantity into a food processor and pour in all the ingredients for the piecrust. Blend until soft, smooth dough forms.
4. Line an 8-inch springform pan with parchment paper and grease with cooking spray.
5. Spread the dough in the bottom of the pan and bake for 15 minutes.
   For the filling:
6. In a bowl, add the remaining flax egg and all the filling's ingredients. Combine well and pour the mixture on the piecrust. Bake further for 40 minutes or until the pie is golden brown.
7. Remove from the oven and allow cooling for 1 minute.
8. Slice and serve the pie warm.

Spicy Cheesy Tofu Balls

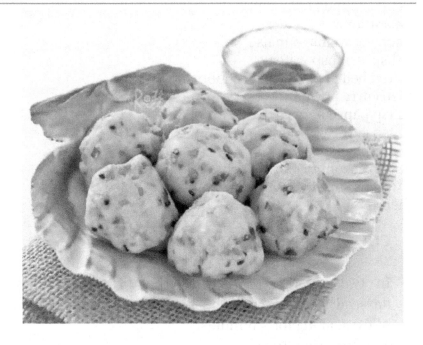

Time: 30 minutes | Servings: 4

INGREDIENTS:

⅓ cup vegan mayonnaise

¼ cup pickled jalapenos

1 pinch cayenne pepper

4 oz. grated vegan cheddar cheese

1 tsp paprika powder

1 tbsp mustard powder

1 tbsp flax seed powder + 3 tbsp water

2 ½ cup crumbled tofu

Salt and black pepper to taste

2 tbsp vegan butter, for frying

Nutrition Facts		
Amount per		
1 serving (10 oz)		284 g
Calories 458	From Fat	274
		% Daily Value*
Total Fat 30.6g		47%
Saturated Fat 7.5g		37%
Trans Fat 0.4g		
Cholesterol 26mg		9%
Sodium 924mg		39%
Total Carbohydrates 33g		11%
Dietary Fiber 2g		7%
Sugars 5g		
Protein 14g		27%
Vitamin A 18% • **Vitamin C** 64%		
Calcium 39% • **Iron** 13%		
* Percent Daily Values are based on 2000 calorie diet. Your Daily Values may be higher or lower depending on your calorie needs.		

COOKING INSTRUCTIONS:

For the spicy cheese:

1. In a bowl, mix all the ingredients for the spicy vegan cheese until well combined. Set aside.

2. In another medium bowl, combine the flax seed powder with water and allow soaking for 5 minutes.

3. Add the flax egg to the cheese mixture, the crumbled tofu, salt, and black pepper, and combine well. Use your hands to form large meatballs out of the mix.

4. Melt the vegan butter in a large skillet over medium heat and fry the tofu balls until cooked and golden brown on all sides, 10 minutes.

5. Serve the tofu balls with your favorite mashes or in burgers.

Spicy Pistachio Dip

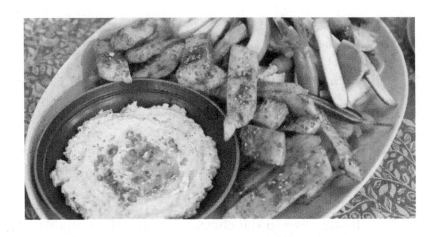

Time: 3 minutes | Servings: 4

INGREDIENTS:

3 oz. toasted pistachios + a little for garnishing

Juice of half a lemon

½ tsp smoked paprika

3 tbsp coconut cream

¼ cup of water

Cayenne pepper to taste

½ tsp salt

½ cup olive oil

Nutrition Facts		
Amount per		
1 serving (3.3 oz)		93 g
Calories 402	From Fat	353
		% Daily Value*
Total Fat 40.7g		63%
Saturated Fat 8.4g		42%
Trans Fat 0g		
Cholesterol 0mg		0%
Sodium 293mg		12%
Total Carbohydrates 8g		3%
Dietary Fiber 3g		11%
Sugars 2g		
Protein 5g		10%
Vitamin A 7% • Vitamin C		52%
Calcium 3% • Iron		8%
* Percent Daily Values are based on 2000 calorie diet. Your Daily Values may be higher or lower depending on your calorie needs.		

COOKING INSTRUCTIONS:

1. Add all the ingredients to a blender and process until smooth.

2. Pour the dip into serving bowls and enjoy with potato chips or julienned vegetables.

Spicy Nut and Seed Snack Mix

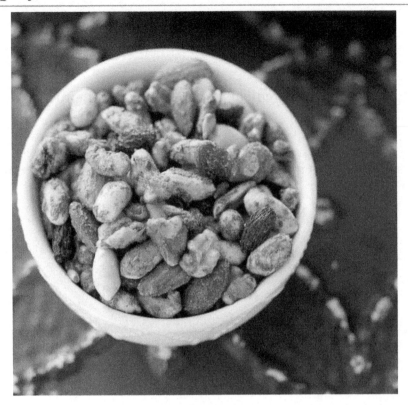

Time: 15 minutes | Servings: 4

INGREDIENTS:

¼ tsp garlic powder

¼ tsp nutritional yeast

½ tsp smoked paprika

¼ tsp sea salt

¼ tsp dried parsley

½ cup slivered almonds

½ cup cashew pieces

½ cup sunflower seeds

½ cup pepitas

Nutrition Facts		
Amount per		
1 serving (2.3 oz)		66 g
Calories 385	From Fat	279
		% Daily Value*
Total Fat 33.3g		51%
Saturated Fat 5.4g		27%
Trans Fat 0g		
Cholesterol 0mg		0%
Sodium 255mg		11%
Total Carbohydrates 16g		5%
Dietary Fiber 4g		14%
Sugars 4g		
Protein 12g		24%
Vitamin A 3% • **Vitamin C**		1%
Calcium 4% • **Iron**		21%
* Percent Daily Values are based on 2000 calorie diet. Your Daily Values may be higher or lower depending on your calorie needs.		

COOKING INSTRUCTIONS:

1. In a small bowl, mix the garlic powder, nutritional yeast, paprika, salt, and parsley. Set aside.

2. In a large skillet, add the almonds, cashews, sunflower seeds, pepitas and heat over low heat until warm and glistening, 3 minutes.

3. Turn the heat off and stir in the parsley mixture.

4. Allow complete cooling and enjoy!

Cashew Butter Roll-Ups

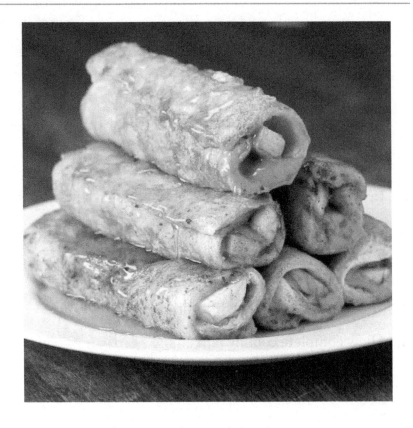

Time: 10 minutes | Servings: 4

INGREDIENTS:

4 whole-wheat tortillas

¼ cup cashew butter

1 banana, sliced into coins

1 apple, cored and sliced into strips

¼ cup golden raisins

1 tsp cinnamon powder

Nutrition Facts		
Amount per		
1 serving (5.2 oz)		149 g
Calories 318	From Fat	110
		% Daily Value*
Total Fat 12.9g		20%
Saturated Fat 3.8g		19%
Trans Fat 0g		
Cholesterol 0mg		0%
Sodium 260mg		11%
Total Carbohydrates 48g		16%
Dietary Fiber 7g		28%
Sugars 20g		
Protein 7g		13%
Vitamin A 1% • Vitamin C		5%
Calcium 13% • Iron		13%
* Percent Daily Values are based on 2000 calorie diet. Your Daily Values may be higher or lower depending on your calorie needs.		

COOKING INSTRUCTIONS:

1. Place a tortilla on a flat surface. Spread 1 tbsp of cashew butter on top and add a few bananas, slices of apples, and raisins.

2. Sprinkle with a dash of cinnamon and then roll up the tortilla over the filling. Seal the ends with some nut butter and make three more wraps.

3. Cut the tortilla wraps into medallions and enjoy!

Chocolate & Nuts Goji Bars

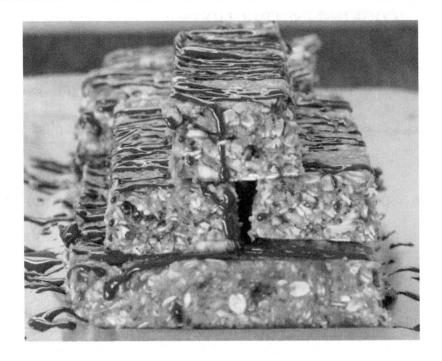

Time: 8 minutes | Servings: 4

INGREDIENTS:

1 cup mixed nuts

¼ cup dried goji berries

¼ cup chopped pitted dates

2 tbsp chocolate chips

1 ½ tsp vanilla extract

¼ tsp cinnamon powder

2 tbsp vegetable oil

2 tbsp golden flaxseed meal

1 tsp maple syrup

Nutrition Facts		
Amount per		
1 serving (9 oz)		256 g
Calories 679	From Fat	548
		% Daily Value*
Total Fat 62.4g		96%
Saturated Fat 22.1g		110%
Trans Fat 1.3g		
Cholesterol 76mg		25%
Sodium 733mg		31%
Total Carbohydrates 11g		4%
Dietary Fiber 5g		18%
Sugars 2g		
Protein 25g		49%
Vitamin A 31% • Vitamin C		51%
Calcium 92% • Iron		23%
*Percent Daily Values are based on 2000 calorie diet. Your Daily Values may be higher or lower depending on your calorie needs.		

COOKING INSTRUCTIONS:

1. Add all the ingredients to a blender and process until coarsely smooth.

2. Lay a large piece of plastic wrap on a flat surface and spread the batter on top. Place another piece of plastic wrap on top and using a rolling pin, flatten the dough into a thick rectangle of about 1 ½ -inch thickness.

3. Remove the plastic wraps, and use an oiled knife to cut the dough into bars.

4. Serve immediately and freeze any extras.

Cranberry Protein Bars

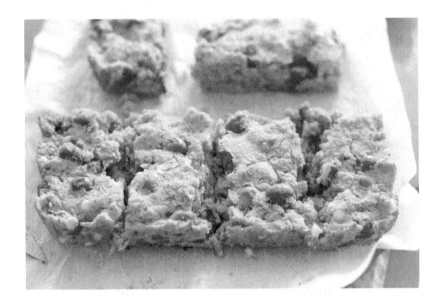

Time: 2 hours 5 minutes | Servings: 4

INGREDIENTS:

1½ cups cashew nut butter

3 scoops protein powder

4 tbsp butter, melted

1 ½ tsp maple syrup

½ tsp salt or to taste

4 tbsp dried cranberries, chopped

Nutrition Facts		
Amount per		
1 serving (11.3 oz)		321 g
Calories 968	From Fat	763
		% Daily Value*
Total Fat 86.9g		134%
Saturated Fat 23.8g		119%
Trans Fat 1.1g		
Cholesterol 77mg		26%
Sodium 1588mg		66%
Total Carbohydrates 26g		9%
Dietary Fiber 4g		16%
Sugars 6g		
Protein 29g		58%
Vitamin A 29% • **Vitamin C** 62%		
Calcium 37% • **Iron** 33%		
* Percent Daily Values are based on 2000 calorie diet. Your Daily Values may be higher or lower depending on your calorie needs.		

COOKING INSTRUCTIONS:

1. Line a medium, shallow loaf pan with baking paper and set aside.

2. In a medium bowl, mix all the ingredients and spread in the loaf pan. Refrigerate in for 2 hours until the batter is firm.

3. Remove the batter from the refrigerator and turn it onto a clean, flat surface. Cut the batter into bars.

4. Serve, and freeze any extras.

Made in the USA
Monee, IL
14 March 2020